# HOW TO
# COPE
# WITH
# CHRONIC
# PAIN

## NELSON HENDLER, M.D.

COOL HAND COMMUNICATIONS, INC.
Boca Raton, Florida

Cover Design by Andrea Perrine

Printed in the United States of America

**COOL HAND** Communications, Inc.
1098 N.W. Boca Raton Boulevard, Suite 1
Boca Raton, FL 33432

10 9 8 7 6 5 4 3 2 1

---

**Library of Congress Cataloging-in-Publication Data**

Hendler, Nelson
     How to cope with chronic pain / Nelson Hendler.
     p. cm.
     Includes bibliographical references and index.
     Preassigned LCCN: 93-70522.
     ISBN:  1-56790-043-7


     1. Intractable pain.          I. Title.

RB127.H4635 1993                    616'.0472
                                    QBI93-839

For my wife, Lee and our

four wonderful children,

Sam, Alex, Lindsay and

Josepha.

# TABLE OF CONTENTS

# FOREWORD

*T*he fact that you have picked up this book suggests that you or someone you know suffers from chronic pain, the kind that hits you the moment you wake up in the morning and tortures you until you fall asleep at night. If so, you're certainly not alone in your misery.

Experts now agree that chronic pain is the third most widespread health problem in the U.S. Its typical victim has suffered for seven years, undergone three to five major operations, spent from $50,000 to $100,000 on doctor bills and stands a better than fifty-percent chance of becoming a drug addict. Incredibly, however, this person's agony has mostly been ignored or worse yet, mistreated by physicians woefully lacking in real knowledge about chronic pain and the devastating effects it can have on its victims and their families.

If you've ever been told by your doctor to "go home and forget it—it's all in your head," this book is for you. Whether your problem is lower back pain, arthritis, migraine headaches, stomach discomfort, housemaid's knee or tennis elbow, chances are you're not getting the help you need if the pain has lasted six months or longer. This book was written to give you that help.

Its author is Dr. Nelson H. Hendler, long a pioneer in the field of pain research and one of the first medical practitioners to differentiate between acute pain (which abates when its cause is healed) and chronic pain (which often defies diagnosis and treatment). Due in great measure to Dr. Hendler's ground-breaking research, the medical community now recognizes chronic pain as a disease unto itself, and over the past few years, clinics have sprung up across the U.S. for the purpose of treating this debilitating disorder. Dr. Hendler is the director of one of the most respected of these facilities, the Mensana Clinic in Stevenson, Maryland, where he continues to lead the way in showing people how to cope with chronic pain and return to productive lives.

When the debut edition of this book was published in 1978, it was widely hailed by doctors and lay people alike as the first complete guide to the understanding of chronic pain. Still the best book on the subject in 1993, it's now been completely revised and updated by Dr. Hendler to document the tremendous changes and breakthroughs that have occurred in this area of medicine in the last fifteen years. In the words of Dr. Hendler: "I hope this book will educate physicians as well as patients and their families about chronic pain. It is my goal to make the problem less mysterious and less frightening by pointing out steps that everyone involved can take to help the pain victim help himself."

Chris K. Hedrick
Publisher

# PREFACE

*I*f you suffer from any sort of chronic pain, you have a lot of company. Low back pain, for example, afflicts millions, while hundreds of thousands of people suffer from arthritis, bursitis, tennis elbow and housemaid's knee. There are thousands smitten by causalgia, a searing pain that often results from a shock to the nervous system; there are also neuralgia victims and those who experience phantom limb pain, which can attack an amputee years after the limb has been severed. This book examines all these problems, along with toothaches, earaches, excruciating migraine headaches and the torturous pain of terminal cancer caused either by the blockage of organs by tumor growth or the out-and-out destruction of tissues by the disease.

Chronic pain can become your master. It can change your personality, define your lifestyle and affect your attitude and behavior toward other people as well as theirs toward you. When this happens, you suddenly find yourself being attacked by anxiety and depression, chronic pain's partners in making you feel bad. These and other related emotions such as frustration, anger, self-pity and fear can cause their own type of pain and trap you in a vicious pain circle. Say your nagging, stabbing pain begins in the morning, so you take some medication that offers a temporary respite. By afternoon you may begin to tense up from anxiety brought on by the anticipation of pain, the fear that it will return before you're supposed to take your pills again. The tension causes your muscles to ache and your head to throb. You begin to feel depressed—your life seems to be ruled by pain and pills.

This book will show you how to escape that stranglehold. It will explain how your home life, ethnic background, social status and even your paycheck can all be components of your pain—and it will teach you how to build a defense against the agony that seeks to control your life.

Coping with chronic pain involves learning all about it, understanding the enemy in order to squelch it. Where does chronic pain come from? How does it start? Can it be stopped? This book will tell you, in terms you can comprehend, about pain and its place in the body's nervous systems, how the systems work and how they send pain messages to the brain. You will see that, unlike other types of pain, chronic pain has no apparent meaning and offers no real hope of an end in sight, whereas the pain of a cut or a ruptured appendix is a useful warning that something is amiss. This kind of pain stops after corrective measures are taken, and it usually does not return.

Chronic pain is something altogether different for which there are no magical cures. In fact, securing relief from chronic pain is hard work, and treatment can be both emotionally and physically demanding. But, as you'll discover in the pages that follow, you don't have to go it alone. There are doctors and other people more than willing to assist you in the quest for what seems an elusive goal—freedom from pain. You will learn that pain messages can be interrupted, halted in their tracks. You will learn that you can stop that pain, and so can your doctor, and that relief is in sight. Moreover, you will learn how to cope with chronic pain through exercises and special behavioral techniques that you can practice on your own to help change your attitude so pain stops being the focus of your life.

Throughout this book, chronic pain is referred to as a disease, not a symptom of some other disorder. This is an important distinction to make and one of the keys to successfully treating chronic pain victims. Sadly, the medical community was slow to recognize this pertinent fact. As recently as fifteen years ago, the vast majority of chronic-pain victims were viewed by most doctors as hypochondriacs or mental cases and thus doomed to a lifetime of suffering with death as their only hope of relief.

Such was the case when my interest in the problem of chronic pain began. I was a third-year resident in psychiatry at Johns Hopkins University Hospital at the time, and my job entailed providing patients with psychiatric consultations. I soon discovered that of all the people I dealt with, the ones I felt most poorly equipped to handle were those who complained of chronic pain.

At the suggestion of two colleagues, Drs. Donlin Long and Tom Wise, I decided to accept a similar position within Hopkins' Chronic Pain Treatment Center. I floundered the first two years, noting the misery of some patients, hearing of the terrible toll pain had exacted upon their lives, while other patients did not experience this same degree of distress. It gradually became apparent there were three broad categories of chronic pain patients: those with psychiatric problems resulting from chronic pain; those who utilized chronic pain to their advantage, and those who responded to the stress by fighting back and working around their discomfort. I also observed the prejudice expressed toward these patients by nurses, physicians, employers and family.

One of the main problems, I learned, was that physicians well-trained in the treatment of acute pain were applying those same principles to their understanding and treatment of chronic-pain victims. This approach invites disaster. To apply the remedies of acute pain to someone whose pain is of a longer, perhaps infinite duration, often leads to drug addiction. Even if the drugs are dispensed by the most well-intentioned doctor, the very end sought is offset by the problems engendered by their inappropriate use.

Clearly, there was no satisfactory diagnostic system for both the medical and psychiatric explanations of chronic pain. So I constructed a preliminary framework for categorizing chronic pain patients in an attempt to understand the problems they experienced. This in turn gave rise to some ideas on how to treat their afflictions. I later found several flaws within that original diagnostic outline, but by and large it proved a useful tool for most physicians. And a screening test I developed is now in use in a more refined form at Johns Hopkins Hospital to help categorize chronic pain patients and determine the type of treatment that offers the best chances for success in each case.

Pain research is much more in vogue these days than it was in 1978 when the original version of this book was written. Since then, scientists have invented new techniques and devices to help pain victims cope, and have learned how to adapt old techniques and equipment to modern methods in this regard. This book examines the most effective of these methods, including acupuncture, surgery, biofeedback, hypnosis and group therapy. We look at the pros and cons of these techniques and analyze what each requires of the patient in an attempt to identify which ones are most suitable to the treatment of your particular pain.

Drugs are also part of the weaponry used in the war against pain. Though most physicians and pain-clinic staff would prefer to see their patients drug-free, certain types of pain can best be managed via pharmaceutical ingestion. How these drugs work is also discussed herein.

You may find your problem discussed in this book, or you may recognize the pain a friend or relative has described to you. Some answers may be of help to you now, or at least sometime in the future. Most important, after reading this book you should be well enough informed to realize that when someone says, "It hurts," the problem may not be as simple as it sounds.

I am grateful to the many people who assisted with the compilation of this book. I especially want to thank Dr. Tom Wise, now professor of psychiatry at Georgetown University School of Medicine, who provided much of the reference material, clinical guidance and moral support I needed during the early phases of my experience with chronic pain patients.

Dr. Donlin Long also deserves a special nod, as he continues to dazzle me with his knowledge and interpretation of symptoms, his grasp of neuroanatomy and his insight into the patients themselves. I have developed a deep admiration and respect for this man and have learned more clinical medicine on rounds with him than I would have ever imagined. Though I am no longer affiliated with the Inpatient Chronic Pain Treatment Center or the Department of Psychiatry at Johns Hopkins Hospital, I still maintain a teaching position within the Department of Neurosurgery there. Dr. Long is chairman of that department and continues to be a superb teacher, a wonderful friend and a great hunting partner.

In 1978 I resigned my faculty position at Johns Hopkins and opened the Mensana Clinic, where a compassionate, dedicated staff and I treat chronic-pain victims from all over the world. I'm proud to say that in our fifteen years of operation we've gained much favorable recognition. In fact, the January 27, 1992 issue of *Business Week* hailed Mensana as one of the eight best chronic pain treatment centers in the country. Our success is due in large measure to the many employees who have remained with the clinic for a number of years, helping to create a cohesive treatment team. For their hard work and loyalty I specifically would like to thank

Andrea Brown (ten years with the clinic), Ann Cashen (fourteen years), Roz Sexton (fifteen years), Chris Kanary (six years), Robert Thompson (six years) and Tom and Carol Fox (five years). Others who are no longer with the clinic but contributed immeasurably during their tenures there include Kelly Silk, Shelly Rymland Redmond plus Lelia and the late James Thompson. Also deserving of thanks are the professionals associated with the clinic who have been most supportive: Sheldon Levin, PhD., Mary Davidson Seiden, L.C.S.W., Carolyn Rousmaniere, L.C.S.W., Kathy Fiedler, L.C.S.W. and Seija Talo, PhD., who spent eighteen months with us as a visiting researcher from Turku, Finland, and who recently won the Volvo Award for Excellence in back-pain research. These people and others have helped Mensana's patients untold amounts, and I am most grateful for their efforts.

However, the real thanks for the creation of this book must go to my patients, who have taught me more about chronic pain over the past eighteen years than all the physicians and textbooks combined. I've seen more than five thousand chronic-pain patients in my time at Mensana, a full twenty-five percent of whom came to us from foreign lands. If this book is helpful—and I believe it is—they are the ones responsible for its success. Indeed, most of the revisions in this new version of *How to Cope With Chronic Pain* were made at the requests of my patients, who urged me to update the medical information of the original while keeping the psychological data basically intact.

And finally, I must acknowledge the help and support of my wife, Lee, and our four children, Sam, Alex, Lindsay and Josepha, who once again tolerated my weekends in the library and forgave me when I couldn't help with their homework or interrupted their other daily routines.

Nelson Hendler
Stevenson, Maryland, 1993

# MYTHS ABOUT CHRONIC PAIN

It's all in your head.

If you ignore it, the pain will go away.

Nobody ever felt as bad as you.

You did something wrong in the past; you deserve the pain you have now.

Pain is the result of abusing your body.

All pain is the same.

You look so good! How can you have chronic pain?

You can learn to live with it.

You feel better if you see someone worse off than you.

Medical science can cure anything.

I won't have to live with this the rest of my life.

My pain is my own.

The doctors don't care.

Pain medicine will help my chronic pain.

# 1

## DO YOU HAVE CHRONIC PAIN?

*P*ain is a subjective experience; it is a personal possession, a private feeling and as individual as a fingerprint. It can be acute or chronic. *Acute pain* is a message to its victim. The brain receives so many messages in a single day that you may completely miss some of the transmissions.

Pulling tangles out of your hair in the morning may cause you some very short-term acute pain. Burning your finger on a hot mug of coffee during breakfast may produce some longer lasting pain. You may twist your ankle while running to catch a commuter train and feel uncomfortable from both the soreness in your ankle and from being out of breath. A hangnail may annoy you all day, or your corns may start acting up because you wore tight shoes. And if your boss yells at you or your children demand a lot from you, a headache may be your reward at day's end. All of these aches and stings and burns are pain messages.

Yet all of these pains are relatively easy to handle. They are short-lived and you don't have to worry about them. You can pinpoint their sources if you notice them at all. The yanked hair, the twisted ankles, the aching corns are all examples of *acute* pain.

Acute pain is generally sharp and short. It carries a warning that has a time limit. It tells you that something is wrong in some part of your body and immediate corrective action is necessary. The time limit can be the instant that it takes to pull a comb through a knot in your hair or the time needed for a broken bone to mend. Acute pain lasts at most for about two months.

Acute pain, therefore, has a protective function. Whether it is the result of trauma (a bodily injury produced by violence or an outside agent such as fire or chemicals) or the result of a disorder of the body's pain-producing mechanisms (lesions on nerves that send or receive pain messages), acute pain acts as a signal for the body to take action.

Because it is a subjective experience, pain is not purely a physical phenomenon that occurs somewhere in the mysterious recesses of the body. There are psychological components as well. These components, no less important than the physical, usually come into plan when the pain no longer functions as a protective mechanism, when it has passed from acute to chronic. Time provides the basic distinction between acute and chronic. While the experience of pain is always subjective and personal, when it lasts through six months or more of periodic or unremitting episodes, pain can be decisively defined as *chronic*.

Whereas acute pain can be readily tied to a source, the origins of chronic pain are often uncertain. And whereas acute pain can be called a symptom of a wound, burn, fracture or collapsed lung, chronic pain is more correctly described as a disease in and of itself. But it is a complex disease, often with an underlying organic cause that is nearly impossible to detect.

For this reason, one of the biggest problems for chronic-pain patients is getting someone to believe that they actually are in pain. Few people who have not experienced pain that persists for more than six months, let alone years, can believe that anyone could live with it that long. The chronic pain coupled with this lack of understanding causes many patients to find life unbearable and entertain thoughts of suicide.

How then do these millions of chronic-pain sufferers get someone to believe them, to give them relief? Let's eavesdrop on a therapy session at a clinic that treats pain patients and focus on a middle-aged housewife...

She sits quietly to the side of the circle of people. Tears are slowly falling down her cheeks. The group leader notices her and asks her what's wrong. She can't seem to answer him, but her face and neck turn red and she sheds a few more tears. The leader once more quietly asks her to explain her behavior or tell the group what she is feeling. She says she hurts. She tells the room full of strangers that the pain is slowly killing her, that it is destroying her life, ruining her relationship with her husband. No one cares about her anymore and her family and neighbors have shunned her because it seems all she can talk about is her pain. The pain is horrible, she tells the group. It's like a knife twisting deeper and deeper inside her neck, never ending. Some heads nod in sympathy and agreement, and her tears stop flowing, for a while.

The woman is telling her therapy group about the chronic pain in her neck that has hounded her for nearly four years. Each member of her group seems to understand, at least a little, for they are all afflicted with their own chronic pain.

Pain is a universally distressing feeling, whether acute or chronic. Both man and animal are liable to feel pain during the course of their lives. Yet while animals are limited to screeching or crying in pain, the vocabulary of pain for humans is more complex. The words that describe pain differ from person to person.

It hurts. It feels bad. It's uncomfortable. It feels like there's a knife slowly twisting in my back. It's a stabbing pain. It feels numb. It's a prickly sensation. It feels like an elephant sitting on my chest. It feels sore. It's a searing pain. It stings. It's simply unbearable. These phrases could all be describing a pulled back muscle, a sinus headache, or an aching limb.

But these are just a few of the phrases used to express pain. They can be describing a sentiment, a physical sensation, or an emotion. It's easy to see why so many physicians fail to diagnose chronic pain or to trace it back to its source: they simply don't know what their patients are talking about. It's also easy to see that the communication of pain can cause a psychological problem for the chronic-pain sufferer. The person with acute pain can point to his broken leg and say what's bothering him, but the person with chronic pain, whose origins are less defined, may not be understood at all by his family, his friends, or even his own doctor. What is so obvious to the chronic-pain sufferer—perhaps a dull ache that continually destroys his sleep—is invisible to others and, what's almost worse, may not be perceived as a serious ailment.

Another problem for chronic-pain sufferers is that their pain generally cannot be measured or tested with readily available diagnostic equipment. A hidden pain, for which no clear remedy can be prescribed, can evolve into a lifestyle for some people. Just like the junkie whose habit dictates a lifestyle of hustling for money, shooting up drugs and then nodding out from their effect, for some sufferers chronic pain can come to dictate when they get up in the morning, what they do during the day and when they fall asleep at night. Many chronic-pain victims have unconsciously hopped on a merry-go-round existence with the hope of grabbing not a brass ring but anything that will stop the constant pain.

If you suffer from chronic pain, you may have hopped on a merry-go-round at your bathroom medicine chest. You were looking for the aspirin bottle. After all, doesn't every doctor seem to say at one time or another, "Take two aspirin and call me in the morning" for almost any illness? In your case, however, the pain did not go away in the morning.

So you took your pain to the local pharmacist and asked him to recommend something. He suggested a commercial remedy slightly stronger than aspirin. Since you told him that the pain kept waking you at night (or sometimes prevented you from getting to sleep at all), the druggist also suggested a mild, over-the-counter sedative. You tried these nonprescription drugs for a while, but they did not work at all.

Without sleep, you became irritable. With nothing readily available at the marketplace that might stop your pain, you decided it was time to see a doctor. You tried to tell him what was wrong. He couldn't see or feel anything out of the ordinary, he said. He took tests, ordered X-rays, poked and prodded and asked you how it felt when he tapped you here and there. He asked you where it hurt. You told him, he listened.

Finally, the doctor wrote a prescription for a pain killer, a mild analgesic. You tried it for a time, took it faithfully on schedule. It seemed to make some of the pain ease up, but it also made you groggy. You went back to your doctor with these complaints, and in his desire to help you get over the pain, he prescribed a slightly stronger analgesic, perhaps with a narcotic base. He also may have prescribed something to make you more alert during the day. But you were so alert, you could not get to sleep at night, so you started gulping down sleeping pills left over from another illness. You ate them like candy. Soon, you were carrying around what seemed like a shopping bag filled with rainbow-colored pills and capsules—but you still were carrying your pain, too.

If you had the time, money and stamina you went to several doctors, looking for one who possessed the magic pill that would give you the relief you were after that very first time you reached for the aspirin bottle in your medicine chest. All the doctors prescribed more pills—to no avail. Eventually you exhausted the best advice in your community; there was nobody left to give you any new ideas. They said they had done all they could for you.

You were desperate, willing to try anything, spend everything. Through the friend of a friend, you were referred to a surgeon who, when you made the appointment, said he might be able to help you, no guarantees. He had helped other people with similar conditions, similar complaints. Maybe he said he would cut something; maybe he told you he would take something out. You were willing to risk an operation, several operations, anything to get rid of the pain.

The pain might have disappeared after the surgeon's scalpel made its mark, but if it didn't, no one believed that you still could be in any kind of pain, especially after all those years and all that money spent looking for a cure.

Unfortunately, in some cases, relief from this lifestyle, relief from chronic pain, may paradoxically bring on another illness—depression. In fact, some scientists suggest that depression can replace physical suffering as a focus for all thought and a determinant for all activity. This phenomenon is called replacement depression, and it attacks people who actually need their chronic pain and to whom the pain has become a useful part of everyday life. The person who has to convince himself that there is a reason he is unable to work, to perform to standards, to have good sex with a spouse; the whiplash victim who heals before his insurance claim is settled; or anyone who has come to use his chronic pain as proof that he's alive—something like pinching yourself to prove that you are not dreaming— is a likely candidate for this syndrome. Take the chronic pain away and you are taking away his security blanket. You may cause him to become depressed.

This replacement depression is similar to that seen in victims of brainwashing and survivors of concentration camps. These people adjusted to their experiences and became dependent upon the routine of abuse as a stabilizing element in their otherwise chaotic lives. Their feelings, activities and even their instincts for survival adapted to that way of life. A sudden change in the routine, even if it led to an improvement, imposed unexpected distress and stress. This stress, in turn, led to depression, or even psychiatric breakdowns. The same holds true for the chronic pain patient who is suddenly "deprived" of his pain. His routine is changed, there is stress in adjusting to a new way of life, and depression sets in.

Chronic pain itself may be addictive. Some scientific studies have shown that brain pathways that carry a great many pain messages come to expect them and carry the chronic pain messages even if they are no longer sent by the original source (like a computer that continues to send a bill long after it is paid).

Chronic pain can attack anyone. How long it lasts and how it feels-dull, sharp, stinging-differs from person to person. Chronic pain is a personal perception, an individual experience, and it is real. Never let anyone tell you "it's all in your head."

# 2

## HOW PAIN WORKS IN THE BODY

*P*ain has long been a puzzle to man. But like a jigsaw puzzle, the pieces that explain it are finally being identified one by one and slowly fitted together to form a big picture.

Pain is a significant event in the body that directly involves all the components of the central nervous system: the brain, the spinal cord, and the acres of nerves. The central nervous system controls the actions of the voluntary muscles, the ones you consciously control. These muscles include the ones you use for walking, waving your hand or bending your head. Pain also affects the sympathetic nervous system, a component of the autonomic system. The autonomic nervous system controls the involuntary muscles, the ones that you rarely think about. These include the heart muscle that keeps blood pumping, the muscles that open and close (dilate and contract) the diameter of blood vessels, the muscles that contract the pupils in the eyes and the muscles of respiration that breathe for you without your consciously thinking about it. The sympathetic nerves go to all the arteries in the body, which in turn control the amount of blood flow to the muscles.

Nerves are key pieces in the pain puzzle. Nerve endings pick up the pain messages that are started by a stimulus (something that incites action). A pinprick, for example, is a stimulus that starts a pain message. The nerve endings impregnate skin, muscle, bone—almost all the tissue that makes up the human body. Hair, fingernails, and toenails do not have nerve endings, which is why you can cut these parts without feeling pain.

After the nerve endings pick up a pain message, it is carried to its final destination by the nerves, which function like a conveyor belt, trundling signals to the brain and back to the site where the message began. There are untold numbers of different nerves through-out the body. The brain alone has billions of nerves and nerve endings. Try to picture nerves as whitish fibers. Some nerves come in bundles, like the bundles of fibers that make up rope, and other nerves may consist of a single strand of material. Some parts of the nerve are coated with a substance called myelin. Myelinated nerves are somewhat like insulated wire; the myelin comes in various thicknesses and acts as an insulator for the electrical charge of the nerve.

All nerves are made up of smaller particles called nerve cells, or neurons. Scientists have been able to photograph these cells through a microscope, and they frequently look like irregularly shaped circles.

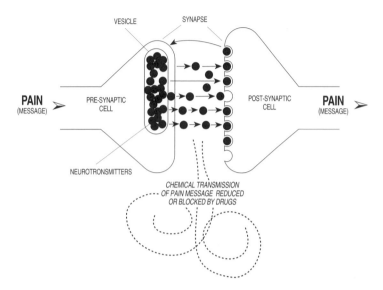

Thousands of nerves throughout the body have been designated by nature as pain nerves. When a stimulus activates a pain nerve's endings, a message of pain travels as an electrical impulse over the nerve fiber from cell to cell along a pathway that takes the impulse to the spinal cord and then to different parts of the brain. The message travels from cell to cell by a complex series of electrical and chemical processes.

Each nerve cell has transmitter and receiver branches, called axons (transmitters) and dendrites (receivers), that help carry the pain message. The message as an electrical impulse travels from the axons of one cell to the dendrites of a neighboring cell. In order for the message to get to the neighboring cell, it must travel over a gap between the cells. This gap, or junction, is called the synapse. It is at the synapse that the pain message impulse is deciphered and sorted, or "zip coded," so that it travels on in the proper manner. After a message is "zip coded," it might simply move on to the neighboring cell, it might stop at the synapse or it might be changed at the synapse.

In recent years, researchers have identified the synapse as the center of chemical activity in the nerves and the key to continued transmission of all message impulses.

There are chemical substances associated with the synapse called neurotransmitters (or neurosynaptic transmitters, as they are also known). Neurotransmitters are stimulated into action by the messages carried by the nerve cell. The neurotransmitter is released into the synapse from the little vessels that hold the substance within the (pre-synaptic) cell. There, the neurotransmitter chemical acts as a messenger itself (the means by which the nerve cells communicate with each other).

When the neurotransmitter chemical is released, it reacts with a receptor, the receiving site of the neighboring (post-synaptic) cell, and conveys or transmits the electrical impulse. You can think of the receptor as a lock and the neurotransmitter as a key. When it turns in the lock properly, everything clicks into place, and the message travels as it was originally intended.

Sometimes, however, the message is changed because of the way the neurotransmitter reacts with the receptor part of the neighboring cell. Things don't click, and the message becomes distorted. In other words, the response of the neighboring cell depends on the ability of its receptor site to recognize and react properly with the neurotransmitter.

Most often, the receptor cell does react appropriately, and the message moves across the synapse and becomes a guided electrical impulse again. The whole process occurs in a fraction of a second and is repeated at each synapse as the message makes its way to its destination.

The transmission process, however, can be reduced (inhibited) or increased (excited), mimicked, or totally blocked—by drugs. A pain message can also be affected by another message traveling along the same nerve pathway, but traveling at a faster speed than the pain message.

Several different chemicals have been identified as neurotransmitters and can be synthesized in a laboratory. These include noradrenaline, also known as norepinephrine, acetylcholine, dopamine, serotonin, and dozens of other less important ones. Different nerve tracts, with their thousands of neurons, contain different neurotransmitters and communicate (innervate) the nervous energy, or message, to different parts of the brain.

To recap: A pain message begins its journey to the brain in a specialized nerve ending somewhere in the body after it is activated by a stimulus. With the aid of chemicals called neurotransmitters, the pain message travels as an electrical impulse from neuron to neuron across the synapses that divide the body's cells from one another, until it reaches its destination in the brain.

Scientists have identified two specific pain pathways to the brain. First, though, the pain message travels through the spinal cord along a single pathway called the spinothalamic tract. This pathway forks at the brain stem in your neck. One branch travels through brain gray matter, the thalamus and the hypothalamus (an ancient part of man's brain). This branch is called the paleospinothalamic pathway, and it is along this route that most dull pain travels. (Interestingly, the majority of chronic pain is described as dull pain, or a variation of dull pain, or a throbbing ache). The paleospinothalamic pathway takes the message to the limbic system of the brain or the portion that controls food intake, sexual activity and the emotions. This helps to explain why most chronic pain has an emotional component to it.

The other pain message branch is called the neospinothalamic pathway, and it conducts sharp localized pain—a good description of most acute pain.

The way pain travels through the spinal cord on its way to the brain is an area of some controversy with pain theorists. A "gate-control" theory was proposed some 30 years ago by researchers Ronald Melzak and Patrick Wall, and its merits are still being debated today.

This gate theory suggests that there is a control mechanism that exists in the "substantia gelatinosa" cells of the spinal cord, a portion of the butterfly-shaped area of the cord. If the gate is open, pain messages will pass through, reach the brain, and make their impact. If the gate is closed, the message will not reach the brain, and, theoretically, you should feel no pain. Melzak and Wall suggest that the "gatekeepers" are nerve-fiber bundles.

According to this theory, small nerve-fiber bundles keep the pathway open, and large bundles, whose signals travel faster than the signals on the small bundles, can close the gate. So the pain of a stubbed toe is transmitted slowly along the small-nerve fibers (designated Delta A and C), and your response of rubbing the painful area stimulates a faster message along the large nerve-fiber bundles (Beta), causing the gate to close and creating a minimum sensation of pain.

The theory also suggests that the small nerve fibers can multiply the effect of the sensory input to different parts of the brain. Such augmented input, the theorists say, would initiate reactive messages from the brain in nerve fibers that descend through the spinal cord. When enough of these small fibers are activated, a critical threshold is reached in the gate system, a point at which another system is activated by the brain. This is the avoidance system, a reflect phenomenon. It theoretically controls reflex reactions (those performed without thinking) to pain—including the rubbing and scratching you do after stubbing a toe, the swelling and itching that accompany an insect bite, crying "ouch," or withdrawing a finger or hand from a hot stove. These reactions can be initiated at the spinal cord without any brain (cordical) involvement at all.

While the gate-control theory has yet to be fully accepted by the scientific community, other researchers have gone on to identify an important component of the body's own mechanism for *controlling* pain. In 1977, researchers discovered that bodies internally produce pain killers, endorphins and enkephalins, chemicals similar in molecular structure to potent opiate narcotics such as morphine and heroin. Scientists had theorized since 1973 that chemicals like the endorphins and enkephalins had to exist, because they discovered the brain has many opiate receptor sites. These are sites on

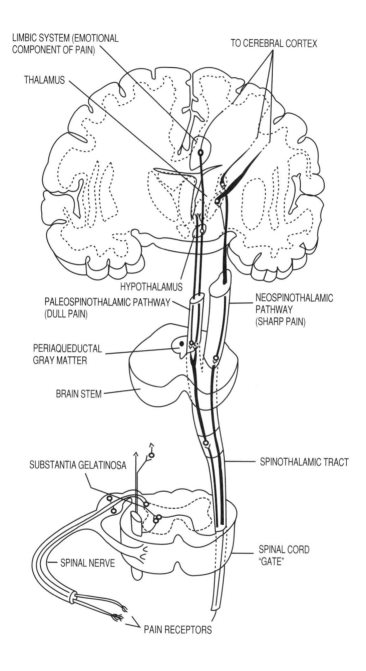

cells to which opium and its derivatives, including morphine, heroin, Dilaudid, Talwin, Demerol, Darvon, and Percodan, attach themselves in order to produce their analgesic and euphoric effects. The scientists (notably Snyder, Hughes and Kosterlitz) reasoned that since such opiates are man-made and not native to the body (yet there are cells in the body that have a specific affinity for these foreign substances) then the body must produce its own opiate-like substances to attach to the receptor sites.

The opiate receptor sites are located all along the spinal cord in the substantia gelatinosa, and they densely populate the paleospinothalamic pathway in the brain. Because this pain pathway goes to the limbic system (which controls emotions), the receptor sites here probably enhance the euphoric effect of the opiates, while the analgesic effect probably begins in the spinal cord.

Scientists have evidence that the endorphins and enkephalins are neurotransmitters, acting at the brain's neuron synapses to influence the integration of sensory information such as pain and emotional behavior.

It is possible that people who seem to feel more pain more often than others may lack endorphins or may have a deficiency of receptor sites. Endorphins may someday be used as a prescription drug to combat depression and schizophrenia. An increase in endorphins may elevate a person's mood by creating a sense of well-being with an absence of pain everywhere in the body.

The perception of pain, however, is influenced not only by the body's chemical system, but also by as many as twenty-seven factors identified by researchers investigating the mystery of pain.

For instance, experiments have shown that a person's pain tolerance varies among different ethnic groups. As part of their heritage and culture, members of certain ethnic groups have "permission" to express pain more freely than other groups, whose members have been taught to act stoically.

Although physical fatigue appears to have no impact on how much pain a person may feel, mental fatigue does seem to lower the pain threshold in some people; that is, they feel more pain sooner.

The *fear* of pain combined with anxiety, also lowers the pain threshold, so if you are anxious about pain occurring, you probably will feel the pain more than if you were not expecting it.

One example of this is getting an injection in a doctor's office. You will invariably feel the shot in your arm more if you watch as the nurse or doctor gives it to you, than if you are distracted by something going on in the office and don't notice when the shot is actually administered.

The Lamaze method of childbirth exemplifies how education, setting and the reduction of anxiety and fear can affect how pain is perceived. In the Lamaze-method program, an expectant mother is taught all about the various physical aspects of pregnancy and delivery. Knowing what to expect of and from the body helps eliminate the fear of the unknown and the anxiety of "what happens next?" The expectant mother is also taught exercises to help her cope with the pain and concentrate on something else. Many Lamaze-trained women, therefore, are able to go through labor and delivery without analgesics or anesthesia because of their reduced anxiety and tension, distraction from the pain and their acceptance of the fact that the pain they do feel is necessary. This is called "psychoprophylaxis," or preparing the person. A Lamaze-trained woman also knows that the pain will cease, and when it does, she will have produced a baby.

How you perceive pain can be determined by your family background, your ethnic heritage, and your own personality (see Chapter 4). If, for example, your family believed that it was not proper to complain about pain, you may have a much higher pain threshold than other people. On the other hand, if your family tended to be emotionally expressive and accepted pain as one of life's burdens, you may perceive more pain than others.

Pain, then, is a *subjective* experience that can be explained in part by scientists and only guessed at by others. Some pain can be relieved or, at the least, tempered.

The experience of pain is not confined to any one part of the body, because pain-nerve endings are everywhere (except in the brain itself). Pain can be packaged as a headache that is continuous and incapacitating. Pain can be a chronic sore throat, or a bursitis in your shoulder that seems to get worse when the weather is damp. Your pain can come from the same organic source as your neighbor's pain, yet you may perceive more or less pain and be more or less incapacitated. These individual differences demonstrate the subjective nature of pain perception.

Pain is a message to the spinal cord and brain. You can be conditioned to continue receiving pain messages long after the source of the messages is gone (Remember Pavlov's dog? He was taught to salivate at the sound of a bell because he was always fed soon after a bell was rung.). Pain is a learned pattern, too, and it is learned rapidly because it is, well, painful.

The important thing to realize is that pain messages can be stopped, by other messages on nerve pathways, or by drugs.

The key factor that differentiates how each individual feels pain is how he perceives it. Think of it this way: There is an old brain twister that asks if a tree falls and no one is near enough to hear it, does the falling tree make a noise when it hits the ground? Applying this to pain perception: if you stub your toe (something that is known to incite pain messages), but your brain is on the blink for some reason (you are on drugs or distracted by something like your house burning down), will you perceive the pain at all?

The answer, of course, is up to the individual, and that is why pain, particularly chronic pain, is so hard to diagnose and treat. While science has discovered many mechanisms and attributes of pain and how to deal with them, the way individuals perceive pain remains a vast field for theoretical answers. It can't be accurately measured, and that makes the diagnosis and treatment difficult.

Many pieces to the jigsaw puzzle of pain are still missing; many, however, have been discovered but have yet to be fit into the big picture.

# 3

## WHY YOU HAVE CHRONIC PAIN

*C*hronic pain is a disease of complex origins and symptoms. It is an indiscriminate enemy that can originate in the muscles or begin elsewhere and attack the muscles. It can assault the vascular system, having originated in the veins and arteries or an entirely different part of the body. It can be neural in origin, emanating from the nerves and the nervous system. Without a doubt, whatever its sources, pain exists on a physical level.

However, there is also an emotional component of human responses that can compound any physical disorder and intensify how much pain any of us perceive. The physical component of pain, which often mimics other readily identifiable diseases, can confound the physician when his initial diagnosis is not confirmed by standard tests. The emotional component can be a mask, too. Depression, anxiety, fear and anger can hide underlying physical causes from even the most astute specialist, who is then apt to give up and label a chronic-pain sufferer's problem as "psychogenic." Such was the cast of a young woman named Jane.

Jane is in her early twenties and enjoyed an active, athletic life until about a year ago, just after she graduated from college. She had stopped her car at an intersection and a drunken driver slammed into the back of it.

In the emergency room after the accident, Jane complained that her neck and left arm hurt. She was treated and released, but the pain persisted. Her physician, an old family friend, gave her a cervical brace that immobilized her neck in an attempt to alleviate the pain there. When the bracing did not appear to help, another physician, who was called in to consult on the case, put her in traction. Finally, she tried denervation (a process during which the nerve is killed by a chemical injected directly into it, or the nerve is severed to kill its effect). This appeared to afford her some relief.

But about eight months later, Jane began to develop pain in her left arm that felt like pins and needles were pricking her. She went to a neurosurgeon who gave her a thorough work-up and found the results were all within the limits defined as normal. She went to another neurosurgeon who also found nothing out of the ordinary, no muscles wasting away, no abnormalities on Jane's X-rays. She went to an orthopedic surgeon. He examined all her limbs and could find nothing wrong. He suggested she see a psychiatrist, claiming the pain apparently was "all in her head."

By the time she arrived at the psychiatrist's office, Jane actually needed her services: she was so deeply depressed that she was close to contemplating suicide. The pain was beginning to rule her life and had taken the joy out of living. On her doctor's recommendation she checked into an institution for four months of treatment for depression. However, the pain in her left arm persisted after her release, and once again she turned to the psychiatrist for help. Unlike the previous physicians, the psychiatrist listened to her and did not try to talk her out of her pain—when Jane said she had pain, the psychiatrist believed her. This alone gave Jane some measure of relief.

The psychiatrist decided to order a new type of pain detection test called thermography (see Chapter 6), and the results indicated that the pain was somatogenic (having an organic source) as opposed to psychogenic (having only psychological origins). The physician then tried a drug treatment on her, one that blocks the slower pain-nerve message carriers from reaching the pain receptor sites. The drug therapy was successful. Jane came away from the treatment with a diagnosis (reflex sympathetic dystrophy) that reduced her anxiety, and with significantly less pain—a minimal discomfort that she could bear and that allowed her to go on with her life.

Jane is typical of the legion of chronic pain sufferers whose disorders somehow fall through the cracks of conventional medical diagnostic systems. While seeking relief, often for many years, these people become afflicted with emotional problems, compounding their perception of pain and perhaps clouding the physician's view of their symptoms and complaints—particularly the physician who is unable or ill-trained to handle severe emotional disturbances.

In Jane's case, the cause of her pain was three-fold. The sympathetic dystrophy in her arm (weakening or degeneration of the nerves that innervate the arteries to the arm muscles) was the cause of her left arm pain. Her acute pain was originally caused by the traumas sustained in her car accident. This physical component then was compounded by her emotional response—her depression at not getting relief, at not finding anyone who believed her complaints and at the limitations the pain placed on her formerly active life. Her emotional state caused her to experience incapacitating pain. These pain cycles that are initiated by trauma and then lead to emotional problems and increased perception of pain are common in chronic-pain patients.

People who suffer from chronic pain are also liable to increase their troubles through the treatment they seek. Often their pain is from adhesions (scar tissue attached to healthy tissue inside the body that forms after one or more surgical operations). If the chronic-pain sufferer is taking multiple dosages of different pills prescribed by several physicians, pain can result from the adverse reactions the drugs have on one another and on the body's systems. In some people, if you eliminate the drugs they are swallowing, you may, in fact, completely eliminate the pain. Also, the anxiety of wondering if relief will ever come can heighten the perception of pain.

That said, let's look now at some of the sources and common causes of chronic pain.

# Muscle Pain

Muscular pain probably accounts for more American health complaints than any other source of chronic pain. It is the scourge of millions, who perhaps one morning wake up and clutch at some point just below the neck and above the buttocks and continue to feel that spot almost every day of their lives.

*Back pain* can be caused by congenital postural abnormalities, or just bad posture, and by neck injuries, like whiplash; but more often it is linked to degenerative diseases of the intricate muscle and ligament structures in the skeleton that allow humans to walk upright. Dystrophy (weakening or degeneration) and disease often attack the back's muscles and discs, which act as cushions. Should discs slip out of place or become crushed, back pain usually is inevitable.

*Low back pain*, located in the small of the back or the axial muscles, is a common complaint. To some degree, this problem is caused by weakened muscles that can be strengthened by exercise. Just being out of shape can open the way for low-back pain. Tension, which can generate muscle spasms, is another source. Low-back-muscle spasms often start with strain or trauma to the region (incorrectly lifting a heavy load can cause such trauma) and then are further aggravated by worrying about the pain, or by any of life's other stresses that accumulate in our daily activities and encounters with other people. These spasms are difficult to diagnose.

Though low-back spasms are common, it is hard for physicians to find evidence that tension and spasms are causing the pain. When you visit your doctor, the spasms may not be present at the exact moment he examines you. If he questions you about your life, you may answer that everything is great, not consciously realizing that you are under any kind of stress or tension, though you actually may be. Once spasmodic low-back pain is diagnosed, however, you will be told that the spasms caused by tension are reversible with the aid of physical therapy (see Chapter 6).

Tension is a stretching or straining of muscles that is often caused by anxiety. This stretching or straining leads to muscular over-activity, producing aches and pains, particularly in the back region. People who often experience a great deal of insecurity, hostility, frustration and guilt may also feel anxious and so experience backache.

Sports often lead to *muscle injuries*, and when a certain muscle is injured time after time in the same manner, that muscle may become subject to chronic pain. Knees and ankles are the most likely victims of athletic injuries. These are actually joints not muscles, but when the joint is injured, the ligaments surrounding them may swell and contribute to the pain. Sprains and strains to muscles and joints are easily diagnosed by a trainer, coach or physician, and treatment usually consists of raising the injured part and packing it with ice. In some cases a tight dressing may be applied to prevent further swelling that could cause hemorrhaging under the skin, and thus additional damage and pain.

*Myofascial syndrome* is a condition of the body's skeletal muscles. (Myofascial refers to muscles and the cellophane-like membrane that covers them). It is difficult to diagnose because there is an absence of neurological or orthopedic indicators for it on diagnostic tests. The pain problems associated with myofascial syndrome often mimic conditions such as herniated vertebral discs, syndromes of the joints in the vertebra, pleurisy and a disease called spondylolisthesis (a displacement of the vertebra producing pain by compression of the nerve root). However, because therapy for this latter group of illnesses is different from therapy for myofascial syndrome, pain relief can be elusive if the diagnosis is incorrect.

Causes of myofascial syndrome include trauma to the neck; muscle tension, such as typists feel in their shoulders after sitting through a long day; and excessive vigorous exercise. In these cases, muscles that normally slide freely against one another are pinned down by adhesions (caused by the trauma). Muscles pulling on the adhesion cause the muscles that are pinned down to go into spasm, since they cannot slide freely.

Physicians can diagnose this syndrome if they can induce pain at several identifiable trigger points in the back. These trigger points are portions of muscles and ligaments that, when pressed with a finger, can cause severe pain to radiate outward from the pressure point. The exact etiology (original cause) is as yet not fully understood by physicians, but they speculate that restricting muscle movement produces the initial pain, and this restriction in turn produces a muscle spasm which pulls the sensitive covering over bone to which the muscle is attached, thereby producing more pain.

Another muscular pain is associated with the jaw muscles that control chewing. This syndrome is named after the affected area: the temporomandibular joint, or

TMJ. *TMJ syndrome* is a perplexing illness because it, too, mimics the symptoms of more readily identifiable diseases. The symptoms that confound the patient and the physician include pain and fullness in the ear (as if the ear canal were stuffed with cotton), tinnitus (ringing in the ear), dizziness or even hearing loss. These signs all appear to be symptoms of a hearing problem, or a malfunction of one or more of the delicate mechanisms in the ear. A physical examination, however, yields only negative results.

There are several possible causes for TMJ syndrome: one is grinding the teeth, a process often associated with the tension that usually occurs while you are sleeping so that you may be unaware that it is happening; another is a dysfunction of one or more of the nerves that enervate the chewing muscles of the jaw; or a misalignment of the jaw due to natural causes, missing teeth or trauma. Treatment involves the use of muscle relaxers, anti-inflammation drugs and EMG biofeedback.

## Neural Pain

*Trigeminal neuralgia,* or *tic douloureux,* is an affliction of a facial nerve (the trigeminal nerve). A bout of neuralgia can be set off by a puff of wind or a slight touch that brushes the face. The pain may disappear within a few hours only to return again, capriciously. Although its cause is as yet unknown, it can be treated (discussed in Chapter 6), using the anti-convulsant drug Tegretol.

*Post-herpetic neuralgia* is the excruciating aftermath of an adult's bout with herpes zoster, the virus that causes chicken pox in children. The viral infection produces lesions on the skin similar to chicken pox marks, but it also leaves lesions under the skin on the nerves of both the central and sympathetic nervous systems. Sometimes when the skin lesions clear up, the lesions on the nerves do not. Large nerve fibers may be destroyed, leaving a greater quantity of the small nerve-fiber bundles—the pain-message conveyors. Therefore, pain messages are sent, and there are no corresponding nerves to countermand them with messages signaling relief. The pain of herpetic neuralgia may be compounded in older people who have atherosclerosis (fatty deposits in the medium and large arteries that restrict blood flow to parts of the body). Dr. Arthur Taub at Yale University, has used Elavil and Prolixin to treat this disorder.

*Neuromas* are tumors that form on nerve endings; they can cause strong and lasting chronic pain. These tumors grow where a nerve has been injured or severed in an accident. Some people are prone to forming neuromas, just as some people are prone to forming keloids, excessive, lumpy-looking scar tissue. No treatment seems truly effective.

*Palatal myoclonus* is another syndrome found in chronic pain sufferers. It is a disorder of the palate or the roof of the mouth, in which the muscles in this area expand and contract rapidly, though involuntarily, in a rhythmic (myoclonic) motion. Other muscles in the head and neck may also be involved. Palatal myoclonus can be caused by a neurological disorder set off by trauma, or by a vascular disease near the brain stem. Sometimes physicians are unable to pinpoint the etiology. Sometimes, surgery is effective.

*Sympathetic dystrophy* is a weakening or degeneration of sympathetic nerves, usually caused by trauma. Pain associated with the sympathetic dystrophy can appear in places that were not affected by the original trauma, as in Jane's case. Causalgia is a general term used to describe pain caused by nerve damage. It is usually a burning sensation.

*Thoracic outlet syndrome* is commonly misdiagnosed, and there are physicians who don't even believe it exists. An injury such as whiplash or a strong pull on the arm may cause the nerves that supply the arm to stretch, resulting in a pins-and-needles, tingling sensation that runs the length of the arm and sometimes into the fingers. From there, the pain may spread into the chest, back of the neck and shoulder blade.

## Vascular Pain

One of the most familiar forms of vascular pain is the headache, in particular the *migraine headache*, a throbbing pain caused by spasms of the blood vessels around the brain. These spasms may be brought on by an allergic reaction to some food or substance, though they are frequently the result of frustration, tension and stress.

Arteries damaged by the buildup of fatty deposits due to *atherosclerosis* also cause chronic pain. The buildup of these fatty deposits can be traced to a high-cholesterol diet or may be the result of an inherited predisposition.

## Terminal Cancer Pain

Terminal cancer pain is different from most other chronic pain *as there is a definable end*, and an easily identified reason for it, whereas with most other chronic pain, the end is unknown.

Terminal cancer pain comes about when tumor growth blocks certain organs and displaces these or other organs from their intended positions in the body. The pain can come from the destruction of organs, bones and other tissues by tumors and from a direct attack by cancer growth on the nerves. Also, radiation, which is sometimes used to treat certain types of cancer, may produce scarring that traps the nerves and produces pain.

## Phantom-Limb Pain

Phantom-limb pain is a bizarre manifestation in which amputees complain of severe pain in their lost limb. It may be caused by the destruction of nerve endings in the amputated part of the body. Transcutaneous nerve stimulation sometimes helps.

## Stomach and Intestinal Pain

*Stomachache* and *heartburn, pancreatitis, gallstones, chronic constipation, ulcers, ileitis, colitis, polyps and hemorrhoids* are all sources of chronic stomach and intestinal pain. Some of these ailments are worsened when emotional problems are translated into stomach pain; others are degenerative diseases caused by the malfunction of a major organ such as the liver or gallbladder.

Improper diet can result in stomachache. Overdoses of laxatives can produce chronic constipation that causes stomachache. Too much aspirin can bring on gastritis, an irritation of the stomach lining. Overindulgence in alcohol can also lead to gastritis and pancreatitis. Too much coffee or any beverage containing caffeine can contribute to diarrhea and eventually gastritis. Alcoholism can cause an irritation of the stomach lining and subsequent pain plus pancreatitis and cirrhosis of the liver. Tension, hostility and pent-up anger can aggravate any of these diseases.

The etiology of ileitis and colitis (painful inflammations of the small and large intestines, respectively) is as yet unknown.

# Joint Pain

*Arthritis* is a disease that afflicts millions and is the most common source of joint pain. It is an inflammation of the joints that attacks hands, fingers, hips—anywhere there are joints in the body. The pain of arthritis can be due directly to the swelling of the joint that exerts pressure on the ligaments and other soft tissues surrounding the joints or from stiffness caused by swelling that limits the use of the joints.

*Rheumatoid arthritis* is a virulent form of arthritis that causes the soft tissue and skin surrounding the affected joints to thicken into deformities. These changes in the muscles and connective tissues (ligaments) are thought to be caused by deposits of lymphocytes (cells from the lymph glands) thickening the connective tissue. Lymphocytes normally are filtered out of the blood, but this process stops when arthritis sets in.

*Gout,* once referred to as the rich man's penance for his lifestyle of idleness and excessive food, now is known to be neither the exclusive preserve of the upper classes, nor the result of eating rich food. Instead, gout is a buildup of uric acid in the joints. The acid is manufactured by the kidneys, and when these organs are impaired, they incorrectly process the acid so it is not eliminated as it should be through the urine. This malfunction can be controlled with a drug-therapy regimen and dietary adjustments.

*Facet joint pain* is an often overlooked ailment but a simple one to diagnose. If your back pain gets worse when you lean backwards; if you experience low back pain that does not extend below the knee, or if you suffer from neck pain that never spreads beyond the shoulders, then chances are you've got facet syndrome. Diagnostic blocks of the facet joint (a joint between two vertebral bodies) will confirm or deny the presence of this problem. Treatment for this affliction involves burning out the nerve that supplies the affected joint.

While not exactly a joint disease, *bursitis* feels as if it is attacking the joints. Bursitis is an inflammation of the bursa (any of the fluid-filled sacs that surround the joints) and can be caused by a strain or trauma to the bursa or by an infection in the sacs. Housemaid's knees and tennis elbow are popular terms for bursitis in the knee and tendinitis in the elbow.

## Headache

Some people are plagued with chronic headaches. Not all headaches are located in the same part of the head, nor do they occur for the same reasons. Muscle tension headaches, which account for ninety percent of all headaches, are caused by tension, annoyance or other repressed feelings that lead to muscle spasms. These are usually felt in the back of the head. Eyestrain from overwork, improper prescriptions for glasses or the need for corrective lenses can also push the muscles around the eyes into spasm. This headache may be felt in the eyes or around the temple area.

The *ice-cream headache* is associated with a cooling of a blood vessel in the palate due to ingesting any very cold food or drink. As the arteries cool, they constrict and cut off the flow of blood to the skin or sinuses or ophthalmic arteries, causing pain. Avoid eating ice cream too quickly or gulping iced drinks, and you can avoid the ice-cream headache. Rubbing your tongue against your palate rapidly relieves this headache.

*Cluster headaches* attack in several areas at once, sometimes grouping around the temple on one side of the head. These headaches are thought to be allergic reactions as histamine is found in the tissue cells on the affected side. Histamine (a substance that causes capillaries and veins to dilate) is released when there is an injury to the skin or membranes, such as a reaction by the membranes to an allergin. Recent articles suggest lithium may be a useful treatment.

*Migraine headaches* are usually described as excruciating. They, too, are thought to be allergic reactions because they can bring on an attack with the injection of histamine into a migraine-sensitive person. Acute migraines may be accompanied by nausea and double vision in addition to the pain which is most commonly described as a high-intensity throbbing. However, at least fifty different etiologies have been described.

Another source of chronic headaches frequently overlooked by physicians is trauma to muscles nowhere near the head—for example, muscles in the shoulder, face, back and neck. These muscles can be irritated by bad posture, eyestrain, a short leg, surgical procedures on the neck or the excessive use of neck muscles for respiration in a person who suffers from chronic obstructive lung disease.

What causes chronic pain? As you can see, any number of factors beyond your control: overuse of muscles, accidents, genetic predisposition, viruses, middle and old age, and emotions you might not even know you are experiencing. Whether chronic pain is brought on by some outside agent, such as a car accident resulting in whiplash or a breakdown of the organs in your body, how you handle the pain and how you accept it or regard it can greatly influence the frequency and intensity of what you feel.

# 4

## PAIN AND THE PERSONALITY

$H$as anyone you know ever said something like "the pain in this tooth is going to drive me crazy" or "it's hardly worth getting out of bed in the morning, my back hurts so much?" Many people have had occasion to voice these sentiments. Whether it's a backache that doesn't go away or a headache that becomes part of your life, chronic pain is an unwanted houseguest—it disrupts your daily routine and demands constant attention. It steals all your energy and becomes the focus of your life. Because of its intrusive nature and demand for attention, chronic pain can change your life, the way you behave and the way you feel. In other words, pain affects your personality—the sum total of your physical, emotional and social characteristics—and your personality, in turn, determines the changes chronic pain effects in you.

The following is a case history that describes how pain and personality affect each other.

Martha is a middle-aged housewife who was happy with her life. Turning fifty didn't phase her; growing older just meant there was more breathing space for her. Her children, who had been difficult adolescents, were finally grown up, decently she thought, and they had all left the nest to make their own way. She was confident she had done her best by them.

Martha's husband had recently achieved seniority in his union, so their financial future was looking good, and with the children gone, she finally had some time to herself. She kept the house the way she wanted and got a part-time job in the local hardware store, run by her cousin.

One day while discussing a sale with her cousin, Martha noticed that her voice sounded different, as if she had a frog in her throat. Her cousin mentioned something to that effect, too. Over the next few days her voice did not get better, so she thought she was coming down with laryngitis. She took to her bed and dosed herself with aspirin and cold-medicine time capsules. But her voice did not get better. Reluctantly, she went to see the family doctor, who, after examining her throat, referred her to an ear, nose and throat specialist or otolaryngologist. This doctor told Martha that one of the vocal cords in her throat was palsied (shaking) because of a degenerating muscle. Surgery would have to be performed if her voice were to sound normal again.

Martha was afraid; she'd never had an operation. She didn't like doctors much, and she liked hospitals even less. But her husband said the sound of her voice was disconcerting, and sometimes annoyed him because he didn't recognize it. After thirty years of living with her, he was accustomed to hearing her speak in a certain way. In addition, customers at the store were complaining that they couldn't understand her. In order to get her life back to normal, Martha reluctantly consented to the operation.

The otolaryngologist explained that the surgery was fairly complicated. It involved making an incision just above her collarbone and attaching one of her good vocal muscles to the weakened one. The idea of the incision terrified Martha; she told him it sounded as if he were going to cut her throat. Despite her fears, however, she went ahead with the procedure and the operation was a success.

After her recovery, Martha's voice sounded fine, just the way it used to. But now she complained of numbness and a burning sensation in her left arm. How could an operation on her throat produce side effects like that, she wondered—and so did the specialist. He told Martha's family doctor that she had most likely undergone a "hysterical conversion;" that is, she transformed her fear and anxiety about having surgery into pain in order to continue receiving the extra attention she had enjoyed in the hospital. Both doctors told her to just ignore the pain.

But Martha couldn't ignore the pain. It was always there. Doing housework made it worse, and if she tried to work at the hardware store, the pain drove her to distraction and caused her to make silly, frustrating mistakes. She complained to her husband, and he complained back to her. He wanted her to stop griping. But Martha couldn't stop griping any more than she could stop the pain. She seemed to hurt all the time, and she hated it and resented the constant pain. She kept asking herself, "Why me? What did I do to deserve this pain?" Then she felt sorry for herself and hurt all the more. She cursed the pain, cursed her husband who did not seem to understand, and ended up cursing herself for having the operation that left her with the pain.

After Martha stopped cursing, she tried to adjust. She appeared to vacillate more and more between hate and acceptance. She stopped keeping an immaculate house. All that bending, stretching, lugging, walking and polishing did not seem to be worth the effort. She did, however, keep the house well enough so that her husband would not notice the difference. She was scared that he might be even more angry with her, aside from her complaints of pain, if she stopped doing the one thing she thought she did best.

She quit her job, though, because her cousin didn't understand her anymore, did not want to gossip with her over coffee, did not want to pal around with her in general because, her cousin said, the topic was always the pain in Martha's arm. Martha had become a complaining nag.

Martha once more went to her physician, and he prescribed some pain killers; but as soon as they wore off, the pain returned. She became bitter and depressed about not having a job anymore, and she was angry at her husband. She was no longer a contented person and did not look forward to doing anything.

Martha eventually went to another physician who took a series of tests. Most of the tests were negative; in fact, it seemed the only thing wrong was that the scar on her left collarbone was hypersensitive to touch. Her left arm and hand retained a normal appearance. Thermography, however, turned up a mild reflex sympathetic dystrophy. Some of the nerves controlling the blood vessels to Martha's left arm and hand had been slightly damaged during her first operation. The physician performed several sympathetic nerve blocks (an injection of a chemical into a sympathetic nerve in order to kill the nerve), and this gave Martha quite a bit of relief. Physical therapy also was prescribed. With the bending and stretching exercises, the pain lessened even more.

Martha returned to work and now does as she pleases again. She's not as happy as she once was, though. She retains some bitterness for her husband and cousin who did not believe her when she was in constant pain.

Martha's pain changed her from a fairly happy woman with a bright outlook on life and a good relationship with her husband and friends to a depressed person no one wanted to associate with—and she didn't care. Pain had become the focus of her life.

Not all chronic-pain patients adjust or react in the same manner as Martha. How a person adjusts to daily, intractable pain is determined in part by his "premorbid" adjustment. Premorbid refers to the time before the person became afflicted with pain; his adjustment refers to a description of what he was like, what kind of relationships with other people he maintained, and how he felt about himself, before the pain began.

To better understand how pain and personality interact, it is useful to categorize, very generally, chronic-pain patients into four main types. These categories, which also help physicians decide treatment methods, compare patients according to different personality traits and behaviors exhibited at different times. For example, a patient might be categorized according to his premorbid adjustment when compared and contrasted to his adjustment to life with pain.

Another factor that differentiates chronic-pain patients is the "chronicity" of their condition—how long the patient has actually experienced the pain, how much of his life has the pain taken over and the activity replaced by his focusing on pain.

For example, was the pain originally due to an

injury or physical trauma, or did it appear out of nowhere one day? Is the pain located in a specific spot or
does it affect a general area that is difficult for the patient
to pinpoint? Onset of pain is still another important
element in the development of a chronic-pain personality type.

A person's environment and the day-to-day circumstances beyond human control will also influence
how that person handles pain. For example, someone
who has a healthy spouse to depend on might notice
pain more than someone who's responsible for support-
ing a family. That person may place his or her responsibility above the pain, shoving it into the background and
refusing to allow it to interfere.

Considering these factors and others, we have
developed four categories to identify the different types
of chronic-pain patients: Type 1, the Copers; Type 2, the
Exaggerators; Type 3, the Mopers; and Type 4, the
Malingerers (conscious and unconscious). These categories are based on observations derived from working
with some 2,000 chronic-pain patients over a period of
five years. They are generalizations and meant only to
serve as a framework to help us understand how a
personality can affect pain, and how pain can influence
personality.

## Type I, the Copers

About half of all chronic-pain patients fall into the
coper category. The coper is a stable person whose life
is orderly and organized until he suddenly becomes
afflicted with a condition about which he knows noth-

ing. He tries to cope with his chronic pain but fails. Soon his time and energy are consumed fighting the pain while his life spins out of control.

Interestingly, in most of the copers I've seen over the years, their pain can be directly traced to a lesion or some other problem revealed by diagnostic testing. Copers invariably describe their lives before pain as "normal" — married, with a decent work record and a tendency to establish and follow a regular daily routine. But chronic pain interrupts the coper's comfortable pattern - and the results are always negative. When the pain lasts between two weeks and two months, the coper acts as if nothing is wrong; he takes it in stride. He may even try to "beat" the pain by speeding up his activity, perhaps feigning a quick recovery and returning to work against his doctor's advice.

He will try to ignore the pain, dismiss it as temporary and refuse to recognize any disability it may cause. He will not allow his family or friends to sympathize with him. Pain to the coper is just one of life's little pitfalls, something to be encountered, then conquered. Basically, the coper denies he has a problem.

However, if the pain lasts as long as six months, it begins to take its toll on this normally stable personality. The coper becomes touchy and angers easily. He has difficulty falling asleep and sometimes is even awakened from deep sleep by the pain. He begins to take painkillers, when before he would rarely put an aspirin in his mouth. His life becomes a little more lonely, he doesn't go out as often as he used to and he doesn't try to socialize with people at work during coffee breaks or other free times.

When the pain becomes entrenched, when it claims from six months to eight years of his life, the coper inevitably becomes depressed. This kind of depression is not a "down in the dumps" or a temporary "blue" feeling. This depression is a serious illness, not just a health hazard but a hazard to life. The coper is depressed because he feels he has lost the ability to be himself. This once stable person now begins to think of suicide as a method of escaping pain. He has lost hope that the pain will ever go away and has refashioned his life around the realization. He may alter his work habits to accommodate his pain (such as a warehouseman not lifting heavy items), or he may quit working altogether. Depression, in fact, often accompanies chronic pain, no matter what the personality type.

Depression is not the only emotional response of the coper, after years of enduring the pain. His emotional expression may run the gamut from anger (a "why me?" attitude) to despair. The coper may attempt to bargain with his doctor, telling him he doesn't care if all his pain is eliminated; he'll settle for the relief of some of it, even though he knows in advance that his request will not be fulfilled.

These stressful emotions strain the coper's relationships with other people. His marriage isn't as happy as it once was, and his sexual activity is kept to a minimum, if there is sex at all. He expresses a great deal of self-pity to family and friends, and the coper begins to think of himself as an albatross around everyone's neck: he's no fun to be with anymore, so he decides maybe it's best if he keeps to himself.

Pills as well as pain become the focus of his life,

and his habitual use of narcotics leads, as it so often does, to addiction: the coper thinks if one pill is good, then two are certainly better, and so on until he is unable to function without the pills.

Betty Ford, wife of ex-President Gerald Ford, is a good example of a typical coper. In the spring of 1978, Mrs. Ford publicly and frankly admitted that she was addicted to pain killers and alcohol. Her previous bouts with bad health were already well known. While her husband was President she underwent a mastectomy for breast cancer. She also suffered from osteoarthritis (a form of arthritis that attacks the bones) that affected her back, and in addition was plagued by a pinched nerve in her neck. She told the press that her neck and back had bothered her for more than ten years.

When Mrs. Ford talked to the public again in 1978 about her health, she said that she was checking into a California hospital to be detoxified, to overcome her addiction to medications and alcohol. She issued a statement to the public stating that drug dependence "is an insidious thing and I mean to rid myself of its damaging effects."

Betty Ford coped with her pain for more than ten years in the best way she knew how. She continued to work and to contribute to her husband's campaign, all the time sustaining this activity with the coper's last resort—pain pills. But because she wanted to restore the life she used to live, she had herself detoxified.

Getting on with life as it was—that's the key to the coper personality.

The coper lives with pain, but never really believes he'll have to do so for the rest of his life, so he does not allow the pain to completely disable him—he retains some measure of control over his life. He is depressed, but he goes on.

After years of having pain as a "roommate" in his body, he adjusts and adjusts well. He may give up narcotics and find he can sleep as easily as when he was pain-free. He readjusts his goals. This is the single, most critical adaptive mechanism for a chronic-pain patient, since pre-pain expectations of achievement are unattainable. If these goals are maintained, then he constantly feels like a failure. However, if he acknowledges his limitations, and readjusts his life situations to suit new, perhaps lesser expectations, he again enters the world of reality, not wishful thinking, and can better accept himself as a "functioning" human being—not a "cripple".

A primary treatment goal for the Type I chronic pain patient should be the reduction of his anxiety about his pain. By reducing the anxiety, it becomes less likely that his work, sleep, eating and sex habits will be affected. By fighting anxiety, the physician also helps the coper to ward off tension and prevent possible resulting muscle spasms that can create more pain. If surgery seems to be called for, it probably should be done, as the coper has a good prognosis for recovery and adjustment following such procedures—better than any of the other categories of chronic-pain patients.

Martha, who was described at the beginning of this chapter, is a good example of a Type I chronic-pain personality, a coper. Martha was well-adjusted before her pain began. Her reaction was to cope, and with the aid and support of a physician who understood her problem, she was able to return to the life she had left behind while she was concentrating on her pain.

## Type II, the Exaggerators

Joan is an example of another category of pain patient—the exaggerator. Joan is younger than Martha, somewhere in her mid-thirties. Joan was never as happy as she wanted to be nor did she ever have enough of what she thought she deserved. Joan dropped out of high school and married a mechanic, more because she wanted to get away from her parents than because she loved him. Joan stuck with her husband through a few joyless years until she could not stand him or his friends any longer. She divorced him and never saw him again.

Joan went home to her parents and was extremely unhappy. She drifted in and out of reality with the help of her parents' liquor supply. If she did not like what was happening during the day—if her mother criticized her for being sloppy—she turned to alcohol for comfort. She decided to do something spectacular before her twentieth birthday: she would kill herself. She thought the easiest way would be to drink herself into happy oblivion and then swallow all the sleeping pills she could find. But Joan's parents discovered her before she could take too many pills and rushed her to an emergency room where doctors pumped her stomach and saved her life.

Joan went back to her parents' house to live. Instead of raiding their liquor cabinet, though, she started going down to the neighborhood singles' bar, where she met her second husband. When they first started dating, he told her he wanted to make the Army his career; after asking Joan to marry him, he enlisted. This did not thrill her, but he was sent to

Vietnam before she really decided to protest his decision. While he was gone, Joan learned she was pregnant and decided to go live with her parents again, since she could not take care of a baby alone.

Her husband returned after two years in combat, physically unscathed and with an officer's commission. The larger paychecks gave Joan some pleasure, and she and her husband and child moved on to the Army base in her hometown, where her husband insisted they raise the family. After several years of peacetime duty, Joan's husband decided the only way he'd ever get promoted would be to find a job where he could travel and showcase his skills to his Army superiors. Joan protested, noting that she was pregnant with their second child.

She hadn't liked raising one child alone while he was overseas, and the thought of dealing with two alone absolutely terrified her.

He started traveling anyway and while he was gone Joan got a prescription from a base doctor for Valium to calm her nerves. With two young preschool children screaming all day, she began to suffer terrible headaches, and the doctor gave her a prescription for Percodan, a narcotic.

A few years later, Joan's husband committed to a permanent position as a teaching supervisor, requiring him to be away from home eight months of every year. Joan's headaches worsened, to the point where she had trouble sleeping. Once again she went to a base doctor, and this time he prescribed Seconal, a powerful barbiturate-type sleeping pill.

But despite the medication and even with her first child in school, Joan's headaches continued. By the time her oldest was in second grade the pain seemed to be continuous and was no longer confined to headaches; now she was also bothered by pain around her eyes and cheeks. She decided that the base doctors hadn't helped her in the last few years (all they did was renew her prescriptions for Valium, Seconal and Percodan), so she went off the base to see another physician. This third physician prescribed a more potent narcotic for her and told her to come back in a few weeks if the pain was not gone. A few weeks later, however, she was in another state visiting her husband.

While she was there she saw another doctor who prescribed something for the pain and something to help her sleep at night—Joan had not told her that she was already taking Seconal. At the suggestion of her husband, Joan went to see yet another doctor who specialized in the treatment of eye ailments (an ophthalmologist). Perhaps, her husband said, the headaches and eye pain were attacking her because she needed glasses. The eye doctor could find nothing wrong.

By now, after seven years of almost constant headaches, the pain was making her vomit daily, and she was dizzy most of the time. Sometimes it was so bad that she stayed in bed all day. That's when her husband came home from one of his long trips and found her in bed crying pitifully from the pain. He called the base doctor, who decided it was time to hospitalize her.

Two weeks later, staff physicians said they could find nothing wrong, yet Joan still complained of severe headaches and sharp throbbing pains behind her eyes. She told the doctors that she also had pain in her shoulders, particularly when she woke up in the morning. After a few more weeks of running tests, the doctors concluded there was nothing more they could do for Joan. They wanted to discharge her. Joan said that although she missed her wonderful husband and children, she did not want to leave the hospital. The pain scared her. She had suffered for so long that she didn't think she could trust herself to be alone—she was desperate. She

started thinking about suicide again, just to end the
pain, because she knew it could only grow worse.

The exaggerator is characterized by two basic
traits: he has a poor pre-pain adjustment and he complains that the pain interferes with his life more than
someone with his problem might expect.

The exaggerator's poor premorbid adjustment
can be tied to a variety of factors: organic brain disease,
anxiety neuroses, obsessive-compulsive personality,
paranoid-schizophrenic personality, dependent personality, hysteric personality, Briquet's syndrome and psychosomatic problems.

The organic brain diseases that contribute to
poor pre-pain adjustment include such conditions as
senility (from hardening of the arteries due to old age or
disease) and drug-induced dementia (aberrant behavior)
that often is concomitant with prolonged alcoholism or
drug abuse or mixing the two substances. Pain is exaggerated by these conditions and seems to be more
debilitating than it probably is.

The exaggerator with organic brain disease will
complain to his doctor that he has trouble remembering
things, can't concentrate, and can't seem to think on his
feet as well as he used to. His family will report that he
is more irritable and has trouble sleeping. He will then
say that all problems are due to and started with the
onset of his pain. Although tests will show that it has
some organic source, the pain seems to be greater than
what such physical injuries or traumas usually should
produce. Diagnosis of organic brain disease can be made
at the same time that the sources of the pain are being

investigated by an electroencephalogram (an EEG, a brain-wave chart) or by X-ray scanning of the brain (a CAT scan).

Treatment for this patient usually consists of drugs and supportive psychotherapy for the family. With the diagnosis, other forms of treatment seem to fall in place. Once the family knows what is wrong with the exaggerator, they have fewer expectations of his performance. If the patient understands the problem, he places less pressure on himself to perform and has less anxiety about what is wrong with him. He therefore has less need to exaggerate his pain and his complaints will diminish. What happens in these cases is that the patient is so relieved to find out that his diminished capacities are due to an organic rather than psychological cause, that he experiences relief of anxiety and copes better with whatever discomfort exists, rather than relying on and even exaggerating the pain to excuse those frightening changes in his abilities.

> Another exaggerator is Corinne, a fifty-six-year-old widow who lost her husband Joe about five years ago.
>
> Two years into her widowhood, when she was feeling particularly lonely, Corinne began to experience pain in her leg, lower back, neck and shoulder. Corinne had always been a complainer—nothing had ever really satisfied her in her adult life. Joe, who died of a bleeding ulcer, was her third husband.
>
> Three years after the pain began, Corinne told her family physician that it was getting worse. He treated her with facet blocks (an injection of a numbing agent directly into the back joints) in her back, and she reported some relief. But soon she was

back in his office complaining of pain in her shoulder, neck and one arm. X-rays revealed nothing wrong in those areas, so the doctor performed some denerva-tions, and Corinne told him that she felt some relief in her neck, shoulder and arm. Only problem was, these pains were replaced with pain in her lower back and leg, and now she had headaches near the forehead.

Corinne's physician administered an electro-encephalogram and an IQ test, as he suspected that she might be suffering from organic brain disease. There were some abnormalities on both tests, so he questioned Corinne more closely about her personal life and recent medical history.

Corinne said she had worked as an insurance agent after her husband died. The job provided her an outlet for her frustrations by occupying her time and also gave her the satisfaction of making her own money for the first time in her life. However, when the pain started, she became less active seeking new clients and this worried her. After the operation she began to have difficulty with her concentration and memory—just about the same time the pain became debilitating. She felt that her business was now in dire jeopardy because the pain made it uncomfort-able for her to sit for a long time in a car, and it was therefore impossible to drive the long distances her job demanded.

During the pain period, Corinne greatly reduced her activity at work. She also became depressed about her reduced concentration, memory impairment and general condition. She was angry and upset that a younger agent was allowed to service her new accounts while her boss gave her the mundane job of typing up reports.

With the information about her impaired memory and loss of concentration powers, and the results of the EEG and IQ tests, her doctor made a diagnosis of early organic brain disease, which he broke to Corinne as gently as possible. At first disturbed by the news, Corinne later claimed she felt greatly relieved. She had thought the reduction in her abilities to think on the job was due to emotional illness, and she actually felt better knowing it was a physical problem.

Her physician prescribed low doses of a mood elevator and suggested she return to work, not as a high-powered front-running agent, but as an office worker. No longer did Corinne or her boss harbor unrealistic expectations of her capabilities. She experienced some residual pain, but no longer described it as incapacitating. Corinne's new-found peace of mind helped her to cope.

Another type of patient who exaggerates his pain is the person premorbidly afflicted with anxiety or depression neuroses (emotional disorders in which anxious or depressing thoughts dominate the personality). These neuroses may surface upon the death of a close relative, divorce, problems with children, financial difficulties or problems with sex. Stressful situations like these that result in a loss, whether it's of a person or possession, often cause depression. Psychiatrists agree that it's difficult to separate anxiety from depression and that generally a depressed person is also anxious. This person's reaction to pain will be immediate as well as exaggerated.

There may actually be a lesion or some form of arthritic change that shows up on an X-ray. But the exaggerator with anxiety neuroses will cease functioning much more quickly than the coper. He will start abusing drugs sooner, gain weight almost immediately because of inactivity and readily complain about anxiety and pain.

A careful history of this Type II patient's premorbid adjustment will help to delineate his problems and differentiate him from the coper. The key to diagnosis is the immediacy of the patient's response after the onset of pain and an overconcern about the pain. Treatment for pain that in part can be attributed to a lesion or trauma can include denervations or blocks.

The final outcome for this exaggerator can be bright if the source of the anxiety and depression can be identified. Medication may be effective, but the best treatment for this type of patient is psychotherapy, designed to help him understand the conflicts in his life that contribute to his depression and how his depression can heighten his perception of pain.

People afflicted with anxiety and depression come from all walks of life.

Peter, a fortyish attorney married to another attorney in the same law firm, is a good example of an exaggerator with a generalized anxiety that contributes to his increased perception of and complaints about pain.

Four years ago, Peter fell down walking to work and ruptured a disc in his back. He had the disc removed and the pain stopped for a time, but then it returned and for three years bothered not his back but rather his shoulder, right arm and neck. Most of the neurological tests he underwent were normal, but one X-ray revealed a degenerative osteoarthritis (an arthritis of the bone that gets progressively worse) in Peter's neck.

His physician performed several denervations in the neck area, requiring Peter to be hospitalized long stretches at a time. To no one's surprise, Peter became depressed. His color was bad; he had dark circles under his eyes from lack of sleep; his face wore a perpetual frown, and he rarely laughed anymore. Peter admitted he was worried. The pain made it difficult to write, he said. It was affecting his work and making him depressed.

Peter's doctor put him on a mood elevator to combat the depression anxiety and help him sleep.

Peter also entered psychotherapy—and a short time later learned that his wife was carrying on a torrid affair with a colleague. He didn't want to believe it at first, but when he found a batch of steamy letters she had written to her lover, Peter was forced to accept the awful truth.

He pleaded with his wife to leave the firm so he wouldn't have to be reminded of her infidelity on a daily basis. But she refused to quit, and Peter's pain got progressively worse. At the same time his sexual activity decreased to about once a month. He claimed that by not having sex he avoided some measure of pain.

After another year of therapy, Peter finally confronted his wife about her affair and how intolerable he felt their work situation was. She agreed to end her extramarital relationship and enter therapy with Peter. After six months of joint therapy with his wife, Peter found that his pain was no longer unbearable, merely uncomfortable.

Peter admitted that it was while under extreme stress at home and at work that he felt most depressed. But once he found a new relationship with his wife and some understanding about himself, Peter also found he could cope with the pain.

Another Type II pain patient prone to exaggeration has an obsessive-compulsive personality, and this trait contributes to his poor premorbid adjustment.

This exaggerator is an inhibited and rigid person

who is overwhelmingly preoccupied and concerned with living by the rules, standards and traditions he has known since childhood. He is conservative and dogmatic in his thinking, meticulously neat and opinionated. Making decisions is almost impossible for him, as every possibility must be evaluated and thoroughly examined in advance.

Perfection is his hallmark. He is attracted to jobs that are precise and repetitive in nature, such as tool and die making, computer programming, watchmaking or neurosurgery. This type of pain patient is usually a steady worker with no financial difficulties or marital strife.

This patient simply cannot tolerate pain or anything else that upsets the perfect harmony in his life, disables him or impairs his control. Even minor injuries affect him to an unusual degree. He's not a hypochondriac in the strict sense of the word, but he share's the hypochondriac's obsessive concern over the threat of pain and injury. His pain usually has an organic basis. It disrupts his sleep schedule and inhibits his sexual activity.

This exaggerator can be diagnosed with standard tests and treated with mood-elevating drugs or surgery. He wants to be cured and will follow whatever his doctor recommends for treatment. Generally, with assurance from his family doctor or surgeon that he will recover, this patient should improve with time and his complaints of pain will diminish.

Herb, a forty-year-old mechanic, is a native of West Germany. He is the product of a strict religious household and the son of a mother who was obsessively neat. He came to the United States about twenty years ago, mostly to escape from the confines of his family and his background.

Three years ago Herb woke up with a pain in his lower back. He had spent most of the prior evening working on an old car for a good customer. The engine just didn't sound right to him, and he had tinkered with it for hours until it made the sounds he wanted to hear. The customer had been calling him hourly, overanxious about the old vehicle, and this had made Herb even more determined to do a perfect job.

That night he slept fitfully, worrying that he hadn't done a good enough job on his friend's car. The next morning, he woke up in agony.

The pain persisted for several months. Sometimes it felt sharp and other times it was dull. In either case, it seemed to get worse in damp weather and when he worked long hours at the garage. The worst days were those when the pain shot down Herb's right leg. This hampered his ability to bend and made him furious that he couldn't look at his engines as closely as he thought he should.

All the tests his doctor ordered were within the normal limits, but Herb continued to complain that the pain was interfering with his sleep and concentration. He also said it was getting in the way of his work and sex life. He said that what he feared most was that it could lead to permanent disability, or maybe even to a bedridden life. It took months before he shared this fear with his doctor, and when he finally did, he added that should he become permanently disabled he was afraid that he would have to return to his parents' home so they could care for him.

Herb's physician prescribed a mood elevator; the pills helped him to sleep at night and relax during the day. He also prescribed electrical stimulation to the affected area (see Chapter 6). As the relief Herb received increased, so did his confidence about the future, and some of his fears about being permanently bedridden disappeared. Finally, his physician felt he was ready for a denervation (the killing of a nerve); this gave him the best relief yet.

However, one source of anxiety remained. Although most of his discomfort was gone, and he had to admit to himself that what remained of it was bearable, he continued to worry about what was causing the pain. He was afraid that any day it could return in a more violent form and never go away.

After repeated assurance from his neurosurgeon and a three-week stay at a pain-treatment center where he learned to relax with biofeedback, Herb began to rid himself of his anxiety about being disabled and stopped worrying about his pain. Without the worry, he concentrated better and went back to work, focusing his attention on mechanics rather than pain.

The Type II personality who is a paranoid or paranoid schizophrenic usually his a history of psychiatric hospitalizations. This person probably is single or divorced or has been separated many times from a spouse, with a work record to match numerous job changes, a poor level of performance and extended absenteeism. He may also have a history of drug abuse and may have done jail time for these problems or even for assault.

Because this type of personality has difficulty perceiving reality correctly, he may view his pain as an attack by hostile forces outside his body. He exaggerates the pain as he exaggerates other situations.

The pain may be the result of an injury or it may have come on slowly. If hospitalized for the pain, this exaggerator will be a somewhat hostile patient, guarded and belligerent, demanding instant service from the nurses and immediate relief from the doctors. This patient can be diagnosed through psychiatric tests and a history obtained from his family.

Drug treatment usually can reduce the complaints of pain, and with psychiatric care this patient can go back to work or return home as a functioning member of the household.

Neal, an unmarried young man who works in a warehouse, is a good example of this type of exaggerator. He injured his lower back in the winter of 1973 when lifting a box that was heavier than he thought. Immediately he felt the pain and by morning it was in his right leg. The company doctor could find nothing wrong but decided to refer him to a neurologist. The neurological examination showed that everything was functioning within normal limits.

After several years of pain in his back and leg and after visiting a dozen doctors, Neal was furious—all the time. He had seen a neurosurgeon soon after his injury and now decided to go back to him. This time he demanded that he be cured and threatened that if he were not, the neurosurgeon might not live to treat another patient.

The doctor remained calm and had a long talk with his patient, after which Neal decided to trust him, to take him into his confidence. He told the physician that there were people at work who were jealous of him and who were putting poison into his food. The poison was causing the back pain. The neurosurgeon then referred Neal to a psychiatrist, who treated him and placed him on a potent tranquilizer, Thorazine.

Neal still complains of back pain from time to time, but he has been able to return to work.

The dependent personality is similar to the exaggerator who has some sort of anxiety or depressive neuroses. This person's poor premorbid adjustment is characterized, however, not by depression or stress but by an unhealthy inability to live independently of others.

A person of this type may have had a long-standing reliance on a parent for emotional support and may still maintain frequent and intimate contact with the parent. On the other hand, he may have been rejected or abandoned as a child and become dependent on others as a result.

If he works, this individual likely holds a position in a protected job. He is probably a passive person, outwardly compliant, and has not achieved a high degree of success as a result of his fear of conflict.

When stricken with pain, this person immediately becomes attached to a doctor and is eager and willing to comply with all the orders and prescription instructions he receives. He may become addicted to Valium or narcotics and will be moderately or severely incapacitated by the pain. He will complain loudly and frequently about the pain and may gain twenty pounds from inactivity.

It can be difficult to diagnose this type of pain patient. The best clue to his dependence is his refusal to take responsibility for his own care. Instead, he will whine and whimper and insist on frequent visits to the doctor, demanding in no uncertain terms that the physician make him well.

This patient also refuses to stop taking drugs. His best hope for successful treatment is the combination of therapies offered at a multi-disciplinary pain-treatment center (see Chapter 7), and more than one admission to such a center may be necessary. The treatment goal for this type of patient is withdrawal from drugs and an increase in activity.

Carol is a middle-aged woman, married for twenty years to a truck driver. Until her accident three years ago, she had worked as a checker in a grocery store. One day on her way to work she hurt herself when she tripped and fell. When she arrived at the store she was covered with bruises from her neck to her lower back. At the urging of her supervisor, she went to the local hospital where it was discovered that she had ruptured a disc. The disc was repaired in an operation, and Carol said later that the pain cleared up in her mid-back. Yet she complained that the pain in her lower back, shoulders and neck continued to bother her.

Before her injuries Carol enjoyed a good sexual relationship with her husband, even though he was often away from home on business. She was brought up in a strict Catholic home and got married four years after high school. Her husband was the only man she had ever dated.

After her injury she not only was unable to work but her sexual activity diminished—because, she said, the pain made sex difficult and uncomfortable, and sex made the pain worse.

Carol asked her sister to help out in her home— the pain also prevented her from cooking and doing the housework. She gained thirty-five pounds after her injury and confided to her sister that if it weren't for Valium and Percodan, she couldn't make it through the day.

Carol's doctor referred her to a pain-treatment center where, though she was a congenial personality on the ward, she refused to participate in the recommended exercise program and was resistant to being withdrawn from her drugs. During the group therapy sessions she said the pain didn't depress her, but admitted that she was upset with her husband and wished that he would take care of her as she had taken care of him all those years he was on the road and coming home only briefly and occasionally. She was angry with him, she told the group, but was unable to tell him about her anger.

The physicians at the treatment center recommended that she have a denervation, which helped her low-back and neck pain. She eventually was withdrawn from drugs and sent home, still complaining.

Six months later she was back at the treatment center complaining even more bitterly of low-back pain. Her "friends" Valium and Percodan once more were a part of her daily diet.

During a group session this time she admitted that she was afraid her husband was leaving her and that all his traveling was a means of distancing himself from her without having to get a divorce. She also participated more willingly in the recommended therapy on this second go round. She exercised as she was told and began to withdraw from drugs. She received another denervation, this time in her lumbar region (lower back) and reported "fifty percent" relief. She said that she could live with that.

When she went home, she succeeded in convincing her husband to join her in family therapy. Nine months later, she was free from drugs, had lost twenty pounds, and her husband had given up cross-country trucking for a local job, which was a considerable help to her therapy.

The group of exaggerators includes a personality we'll call the histrionic. Nearly ninety-five percent of this personality type are female and they display overdramatic, over-theatrical speech and behavior.

The histrionic person does not form long-term relationships and may, in fact, have a string of divorces or one-night stands as part of her medical history. This person exaggerates her pain verbally rather than in how she perceives it. She uses wild and excessive adjectives. If hospitalized, she rarely looks ill; rather she looks as though she just stepped out of a hairdresser's salon. She also wears revealing or sexy clothing.

This type of pain-patient personality has a need to be the center of attention and uses her looks and an over-dramatization of her circumstances to fulfill this need. Her pain is a perfect device for manipulating family, friends and physician.

When trying to diagnose this type of patient, the doctor will discover some evidence of an organic source for the pain, yet he will not find any signs of depression or anxiety on psychological tests.

This exaggerator needs any and all treatment that the pain-treatment center can offer. Efforts must be made to alter the patient's response to chronic pain, using behavior modification, group therapy and low doses of mood-affecting drugs. Surgical procedures, other than denervation, probably will not help her because of her personality quirks. Indeed, surgery might just give rise to more drama and more expression of pain. By keeping the patient a patient, she remains the center of attention.

Linda is an example of a histrionic personality whose pain turns her into an exaggerator-type chronic-pain patient. She is a thirtyish housewife, married three times, who complains of pain in her shoulders that radiates down to her chest. The pain gradually developed over the last three years, and she says it is worse when she moves things or lifts her arms. Both a neurosurgeon and an orthopedic surgeon examined her and were unable to find anything wrong.

When the pain first started, her family physician prescribed Valium and then Percodan when it failed to "ease up." After a battery of tests failed to reveal the cause of Linda's pain, he suggested she see a psychiatrist.

Linda told the psychiatrist that she was beginning to hate all doctors. They didn't seem to understand that the pain was unbearable and excruciating to the point of being disastrous to her life. However, she also remarked that she had no trouble falling asleep, that she was not depressed and that the pain had not affected her incredibly wonderful sex life one iota.

Meanwhile, the psychiatrist noted that Linda always showed up for her therapy sessions dressed as if she were going to a formal dance, wearing excessive evening makeup and low-cut blouses or revealing shirts. And she never failed to compliment the doctor on his abilities, saying she was certain he would help her get rid of the pain.

Linda also told the therapist that her husband, a successful businessman who traveled a lot, bought her every luxury imaginable and even took her with him to other cities so she could see doctors there about her pain. She admitted that when her husband was home, she would ask him to rub her neck and this action seemed to ease the pain. At one session that her husband attended, he told the therapist he felt sorry for Linda because she always seemed to be in so much pain, and that he now stayed home more often to be with her.

Linda entered a pain treatment center. She refused to give up Percodan although she agreed to switch from Valium to a mood elevator. She also tried a transcutaneous stimulator (see Chapter 6). But after two months she continued to complain that she was in pain, that the new medications were not helping her and the stimulator was more of an irritant than a soother. She was released, but several months later she returned to the treatment center, where once again she refused to be withdrawn from Percodan; the staff even suspected that somehow she was hoarding other narcotics smuggled in by friends. Again she left the center but continued with group therapy once a week.

After several months, Linda began to comply with some of the suggestions that the group and her psychiatrist made, and she participated in physical therapy. She began to go out more with her husband, even though the pain, she said, hurt like the devil.

With the help of her therapy, she eventually changed her attitude and now uses her story of triumph over the pain as a way of impressing all her friends, or manipulating them, and thus eliciting their approval of her new behavior—being pain free.

There is another Type II personality who does not exactly exaggerate his pain. This person is absorbed in his pain and fascinated by it, much as someone is fascinated or absorbed by a glowing fire. This person is a victim of what psychiatrists call Briquet's syndrome.

Before the onset of pain, this Type II personality has already shown that he does not adjust well to life's stresses. He has a long history of not feeling well, of having headaches and fatigue, anxiety, sexual difficulties and bowel problems.

The patient is usually a woman who has had many divorces or broken engagements. Chronic pain takes her by surprise. It usually is general and vague and difficult to describe in words to the doctor.

The onset of pain often sends her to bed—where, if possible, she remains. The pain does not interfere with her sleep, but her sexual activity is diminished. She starts abusing any pill she can lay her hands on, including laxatives.

Physicians can diagnose Briquet's syndrome by using a check list. In most cases the patient can identify at least twenty-five symptoms that she is suffering from in a list of fifty-five, yet the symptoms have never been diagnosed. By the age of thirty-five, she will also have a long and complicated medical history that matches the list of symptoms.

Some of the symptoms that the Briquet's syndrome patient will claim to suffer from (besides vague pain) include: feeling sickly most of her life, headaches, blindness, unconsciousness, fits, convulsions, amnesia, deafness, hallucinations, fatigue, lump in the throat, fainting spells, visual blurring, weakness, thirstiness, palpitations, chest pain, dizziness, appetite loss, weight loss, nausea, diarrhea, constipation, menstrual cramps, menstrual irregularities, frigidity, back pain, joint pain, nervousness and general depressed feelings. (The physician should ascertain whether or not the patient consulted a doctor about the symptoms she claims, so he can determine if they should count toward diagnosis).

Because this patient is plagued by a variety of problems and frequently complains about the intensity of the pain associated with each one, her treatment is usually not directed at her symptoms but at teaching her to deal or cope with reality. This Type II personality should never be challenged about the validity of any of her symptoms or the intensity of her pain (even if it seems that the patient is a malingerer without any actual pain). Treatment can range from the use of placebos (sugar pills) to family therapy, group therapy, electroconvulsive therapy (shock treatment) or sleep therapy. Hospitalization in a pain-treatment center where a range of these therapies is offered can be beneficial to this type.

However, unless the treating physician convinces the patient that he believes her pain is real, therapy probably will fail. A Briquet's syndrome patient takes a lack of belief as a challenge—and she probably will not get well.

Paula is a fifty-three-year-old patient with Briquet's syndrome who also suffers from chronic pain in her shoulder and neck and occasional severe headaches. Most of the tests performed on her indicate that she is a healthy woman, although she does show some signs of osteoporosis (a softening of the bones, usually due to old age).

Paula said the onset of her pain was gradual, that it made it difficult for her to fall asleep and was interfering with her work as an interior decorator. She had no sex life to speak of before the pain, so this was not a factor.

Paula's medical record was as thick as the New York City telephone book. She'd been hospitalized more than forty times, had three face-lifts, reconstructive surgery on her jaw, a gallbladder removal and a hysterectomy all before the age of forty. Her record also listed numerous emergency room visits for sprains and broken bones sustained during unexplained falls. She was taking almost every over-the-counter medication on the market, including massive doses of multiple vitamins, and she was also ingesting prescription drugs, including thyroid medication, a diuretic and amphetamines for her multiple crash diets.

When the pain first started bothering her on the job, she visited three doctors, who only glanced at her medical records and told her it was all in her head. Even her son, a physician, said he did not believe that she was in "real" pain.

Paula was finally referred to a therapist who believed her pain and suffering were real. He took her off most of her vitamins and all the prescription drugs and gave her a transcutaneous stimulator (a device to block pain; see Chapter 6).

Within three months, Paula reported that the pain was under control. She stopped seeing the psychotherapist at this time and joined a church that advocated a holistic medicine philosophy— combining medicine with religious faith. Because the holistic people all said they believed in her pain and understood her problems, it wasn't long before her pain completely vanished.

When psychosomatic disorders contribute to the poor premorbid adjustment of an exaggerator, the first thing the patient will tell the doctor is that he is high-strung. He will also have a history of marital discord, sexual difficulties, financial disasters, tension, anxiety and nervousness. He will cite the pressure he's under at home and work as the source of all his problems, and he'll gripe that he has no time to relax or take up a hobby. He'll describe his pain as a tightness in the neck or shoulder muscles and he might also suffer from facial or low-back pain, or headaches over his eyes. His pain developed slowly so no accident or trauma can be pinpointed as having caused it. As usual, the pain makes falling asleep difficult and it interferes with sex.

The nervous tension this patient feels generally translates into physical tension, and this translates into pain. Heat and massage may relieve the pain, as will certain neurolytic drugs by reducing his anxiety. Supportive psychotherapy is also useful for this type of patient, in particular that which involves other family members.

> Mary is a forty-two-year-old woman who grew up feeling the effects of the Depression. Her parents constantly reminded her of the sacrifice they made to bring her into the world. Her husband, a construction worker, had been laid off several months every year for the last six years. To make ends meet, she took a job as a waitress.
>
> Mary started having facial pain under her cheekbones that radiated toward her ear and even bothered her jaws at times. After waiting four years, she finally decided she could see a doctor.
>
> She told the physician about the facial pain as well as the pain in her neck and shoulders. She admitted that she felt a great deal of tension at home from bickering with her husband and at work from her customers. She told him she had trouble sleeping at night but the pain did not interfere with her sex life. She had visited a local emergency room several years before, where she received prescriptions for Darvon and Librium that gave her some relief.
>
> After listening to Mary's symptoms, the physician suggested she see a dentist, something she hadn't done since her husband began his periodic layoffs. The dentist diagnosed Mary as having temporomandibular joint syndrome. Her physician then made her stop taking the Darvon and Librium drugs. Within two weeks her pain was diminished.

Nevertheless, the dentist urged Mary to enter the hospital to have her bite repositioned, for it was so severely out of line that he believed it probably contributed to her discomfort. During her three-week hospital stay, Mary underwent dental surgery and learned how to reduce the tension by relaxing her bite. Over time, Mary's neck and shoulder pain virtually vanished—as did the tension she'd been feeling.

## Type III, the Mopers

The third category of patient who experiences chronic pain in his own peculiar way is known as the moper. This person resembles Type I (the coper), except the source of his pain is unknown, a condition that fills him with anxiety and fear and causes him to mope and fret about what possibly could be wrong with him.

The moper is not known to be a complainer, and this can irritate and frustrate even the most capable physician, who simply cannot find the cause of his patient's discomfort. He is often tempted to refer the moper to a psychiatrist. However, if he examines the patient's premorbid adjustment, he will find him to be a stable personality who apparently has nothing to gain from chronic pain. Nor is the moper known to be a manipulator who might use the pain as a means of getting attention.

Kent is a middle-age man who works as production supervisor at a paint manufacturing company. He has been married to the same woman for more than thirty years and has two children. For six years Kent complained of pain on the left side of his chest near his nipple and under his ribs. His family doctor ran tests for pancreatitis, arthritis and neuralgia, and they all came back negative. The doctor even tried administering a local anesthetic, but Kent reported no effect except some numbness at the injection site. The pain continued to haunt him, always striking in the same place though with varying degrees of intensity.

Kent was eventually referred to a psychiatrist, who noted that he had a good pre-pain adjustment, a solid marriage, a job he claimed to like. His children were well-adjusted, and he enjoyed a few leisure-time activities such as hunting. Kent did tell the psychiatrist that he sometimes had trouble falling asleep because he couldn't stop wondering if he had cancer and no one would tell him. Furthermore, when he did manage to find slumber, the pain would often wake him up again. This had been going on three or four nights a week for the past three years.

Throughout his years of pain, Kent managed to remain free from drug addiction, though he admitted it wasn't easy. He tried to kill the pain with aspirin, but it didn't help much, and lately the constant ache had been making him depressed. As a result, he was having trouble at work, and at home he found he didn't have much interest in sex anymore. In general, life did not seem pleasant. He even found that hunting, his favorite sport, no longer held any interest for him because he couldn't concentrate on what he was doing.

Then, during a visit to a neurosurgeon, an office nurse said she felt a swollen nodule under Kent's rib on the side of his chest. The neurosurgeon detected nothing, nor did an orthopedic surgeon who was called in as a consultant. Kent's psychiatrist, however, with the aid of thermography, detected an area of pain in the place Kent said ached constantly. The area was injected with steroids, and the pain disappeared within two days.

Three months later, Kent's depression was history, while his interest in sex, hunting and work returned.

## Type IV, the Malingerers (Conscious and Unconscious)

This final group of patients includes people who truly have no pain. Instead, they use the memory of some previous pain to describe their current ("imaginary") discomfort.

Some Type IV patients out-and-out lie about what they feel. They say they're in pain, knowing full well they're not. They are "conscious malingerers."

Then there are those who truly can't perceive reality correctly. These unfortunate folks have either suffered severe emotional trauma associated with injury or are afflicted with a psychiatric disease that distorts the world around them. They may say they're in pain when strictly speaking they're not—but the pain to their altered perception is nonetheless real. We have labeled this group "unconscious malingerers."

Conscious malingerers pretend to be in pain to get what they want. Unconscious malingerers, on the other hand, have some legitimate psychological reason for their pain; there is no malicious intent behind their complaints. It is essential for the physician to determine which type of malingerer he is dealing with, conscious or unconscious, before prescribing treatment.

The person who unconsciously uses his "pain" has "converted" the problem into "pain." Conversion is an unconscious defense mechanism that some people use to protect themselves from life's stresses, particularly those they perceive as overwhelming or unacceptable. However, pain is rarely, if ever, used as a "conversion" symptom, since it is not visible to others. You can't get attention from something that is invisible.

Another type of patient who fits into this fourth category suffers from delusional thinking. The pain in this case is incorrectly perceived. This misperception is neither conscious nor unconscious; rather, it is a manifestation of an inability to correctly sort through one's thoughts and feelings. True malingering, on the other hand, is a conscious effort to deceive someone such as a family member, an organization or business, or an insurance company.

Surgeons in particular should beware of Type IV patients; they may convince the doctor that surgery is important and desirable when it is actually the worst thing that could be done for or to them. Malingerers can be difficult to identify, especially delusionals, because these delusions are real to the person with a thinking disorder. (It's not uncommon for an exaggerator to be mistargeted as a malingerer. But there is usually an organic lesion or obscure disease affecting the exaggerator, which thorough testing should eventually identify.)

How do you determine whether a person is malingering? Once again, you look at the premorbid adjustment.

The malingerer is a person who has tried to deceive other people all his life. He may have an arrest record or a history of drug addiction. If he is in constant financial trouble, he may see malingering as a way to help him out of his problems by qualifying him to collect unemployment insurance, Social Security disability payments or workman's compensation. Yet, it is hard to pick out a malingerer from past history alone, as he is more prone to fake an illness when circumstances call for it, when he sees sickness or pain as a way out of a sticky situation. He may view his deception as self-preservation rather than a dishonest way of getting attention or easy money.

Certain family and environmental situations may also propel someone along the path to malingering. For example, a person who comes from a poor family, especially a poor large family, may resort to malingering to escape responsibilities or duties he doesn't like.

A conscious malingerer usually makes a great show of his "disability," but he's also liable to blow his cover at some point by limping on the wrong leg or forgetting which arm is suppose to be injured. Pain, therefore, is the ideal symptom for the malingerer to adopt, as there is no way to measure it, and the physician can only proceed on the basis that his patient is telling the truth.

There *are* clues, however, that a doctor can look for if he suspects a patient of malingering. If upon close examination there is no muscle atrophy in a limb the patient claims he never uses, or if the patient's condition doesn't get appreciably better or worse over a period of time, chances are there's a malingerer at work.

A malingerer might also reveal himself to a nonjudgmental, unbiased doctor by his reluctance to answer questions or submit to examinations. Consequently, the astute physician who suspects possible malingering will engage the patient in conversation as much as possible, urging him to talk about his fears, problems and anything else concerning his treatment.

The doctor should look for inconsistencies in the patient's attitude and behavior. Is he able to pursue his hobbies even though he no longer works or maintains his household responsibilities? Are his symptoms consistent from one appointment to the next? Did he contact his attorney before submitting to medical treatment? One of these factors by itself might not mean much and probably is not conclusive, but taken together, these clues just may spell, "malingerer."

Obviously, treating this type of patient presents the physician with a difficult challenge. Of course, surgery won't help and therapy most likely will also be useless, although some family therapy might be in order. Benign neglect, without confronting the patient with his fakery, is a possible course of action, though not one most doctors would want to use.

Surprisingly, even a cash settlement may be ineffective in curing the malingerer, especially if he has found his pain or condition useful on the home front.

> Ron is a thirty-five-year-old janitor, married with four children. He's not particularly fond of his job in a factory; in fact, most days he's bored and resentful that he has to work the early shift. Ron has always hated getting up before the crack of noon.
>
> One day soon after he arrived at work and punched in, Ron lifted a heavy box to toss into the trash bin and suddenly felt a pain in his lower back. He immediately went to his supervisor and told him he'd strained his back.
>
> Ron's supervisor sent him to the company doctor, who told Ron to go home immediately and spend a couple of days in bed, just resting. While he was home, Ron called his cousin, an attorney, because

his union steward told him the company ought to do something for him beyond sending him home for a few days. After talking with his cousin, Ron started to put together some information that he could use to get workman's compensation.

Ron told the Workmen's Compensation Board that the pain in his back was so bad that he was no longer able to work and couldn't even have sex with his wife anymore. The board granted him compensation, as did Social Security administrators, whom he had also contacted within a day of being injured. Suddenly, Ron was making more money than his janitor job had ever provided. With all that loot coming in and plenty of time on his hands, Ron decided to do something constructive and enrolled in a course to learn appliance repair.

Meanwhile, he had to return to the company doctor for periodic physical examination by order of the Workmen's Compensation Board. The doctor listened to Ron's complaints of pain and noted that he was able to lift his legs while seated but not when he was lying down. The doctor sent him to another board physician for a psychiatric evaluation, which showed him to be a passive person with some anxieties and depression. The board decided Ron should return to work.

At the same time, the factory's insurance company hired an investigator to spy on Ron in an effort to determine whether or not his claim should be paid. Using hidden cameras, the insurance people found that he could lift heavy boxes when no one was around and that he also rode a motorcycle when he thought no one was watching. Ron did not seem to be in any pain when he was lifting those boxes or riding the motorcycle. He was asked to see the psychiatrist once more.

Because the doctor seemed sympathetic, Ron tearfully admitted that it was not so much that he was in pain but that he could never handle the work load that was assigned to him, and he was afraid his fellow workers would laugh at him and think he was a sissy if they knew. Ron also admitted that he didn't have sex with his wife anymore because she had gained about fifty pounds after her last pregnancy and had never taken it off. Fat people always repulsed him, he said.

After counseling, Ron agreed to undergo psychotherapy with his wife and participate in vocational rehabilitation. Soon he was trained for a new job and his wife lost forty pounds. At that point, Ron quit collecting disability payments and went to work again—in an appliance store.

Ron was a classic malingerer who used his pain to escape a stressful situation at work. He also found it was useful at home as a weapon against his wife's "repulsive" obesity. Once the home and work situations were resolved to his satisfaction, his pain was resolved as well.

The Type IV personality whose pain is due to conversion or delusion is not as easy to help. There are so few cases of this type personality that doctors find it difficult to properly diagnose the symptoms.

Conversion is not an easy process to understand and can mask other psychiatric or organic ailments. Even people who are considered "normal" in every way may experience conversion symptoms during overwhelmingly stressful times—especially after a traumatic incident. For example, the wife who is driving the car when there is an accident that kills her passenger—her husband—may convert her grief and guilt into an excruciating back or neck pain. There is no typical premorbid adjustment for the personality that converts life stresses or traumas into pain. This is because conversion is usually an unexpected consequence—it represents a method of coping. Because it is an unconscious event, the person believes and is convinced the pain is real. Indeed, this is not to say the pain is imaginary for there is no such thing. But what happens with the patient who experiences conversion is that he perceives pain, though it is strictly related to an emotional event and not to any organic source. The pain is real in that it probably hurts, but it is only real as long as the patient needs it as a coping mechanism. Treatment for this kind of pain includes the use of psychotherapy an mood-elevating drugs. In extreme cases, electroconvulsive therapy might be prescribed.

Frieda is a fortyish computer programmer, a fussbudget who demands perfection from herself in all phases of her life. She was divorced abruptly after a ten-year marriage because she felt that she and her husband were incompatible.

About one month after an auto accident, Frieda started complaining about a pain at the back of her head. She also claimed she was losing her ability to concentrate and calculate figures, a necessary part of her job.

She went to a doctor who administered a brainwave (EEG) and several other neurological tests and found them all to be normal. While taking her history, the doctor learned that she had suffered a depression after her divorce for which she briefly went into therapy.

Frieda admitted to her physician that she was compulsive about her work, but said the job demanded the utmost attention to detail. She told him she was depressed most of the time now that she had the pain, and she had trouble falling asleep.

The doctor thought Frieda's problems could have resulted from the concussion she suffered in the accident. He prescribed some mood elevators for her, but Frieda still didn't feel well, and she quit work because she claimed her inability to concentrate made it impossible to run programs properly.

After three months of drug therapy, Frieda reported an improvement in concentration and revealed that she had gone back to work part time. But she was still too afraid of making mistakes to return to full-time duty.

During her part-time employment, Frieda tried to sue the person who had hit her car. Unfortunately, however, she discovered he was uninsured and had fled the state to avoid arrest for a host of other misdemeanors (he was out on bail at the time of the car accident). Frieda told her doctor that she knew she would never collect from him, and she felt that both he and the insurance company had cheated her. The doctor suggested she try psychotherapy, and Frieda agreed.

During therapy sessions it came out that Frieda had always been afraid she would die in an auto accident and so was terribly shaken by her recent one. However, the catharsis of her admission did not help get rid of her headaches. Then, during one of her sessions after a year in therapy, Frieda recalled an incident from childhood, when her mother struck her on the back of her head because she had refused to tie her shoes. She immediately realized that the blow she had received from her mother felt exactly like the blow she had suffered during the car accident. Furthermore, she remembered the frustration she had felt as a child because she was unable to strike back at her mother for what she considered unjust punishment. Those same feelings surfaced toward the driver who had smacked her car and fled without paying for damages. Just as Frieda had wanted to kill her mother for the blow on the head, she also wanted to kill the driver for destroying her car and her ability to concentrate, a vital part of her life. In front of her psychiatrist, Frieda burst into tears, and by the following week, her headaches had virtually disappeared.

Chronic pain can be extremely difficult to diagnose and treat, for it's as diverse and complex as the personalities of the people afflicted by it.

No matter what causes the pain (although it usually has an organic basis), the patient's personality has an overwhelming effect on treatment and the rate of recovery. If the patient really wants to get better and return to the way life was before the pain, there's a good chance for success. But if the patient discovers a special use for the pain, the most sophisticated drugs and devices may not alleviate it.

All pain (except in the case of the conscious malingerer) is perceived as real to the person who is suffering from it. This must be accepted by everyone involved in the treatment process—the physician as well as the patient.

The realization that plenty of other people in the world share your problem and complaints may make it easier for you to cope with chronic pain. Indeed, knowing that even the coper has a difficult time adapting to it and living with it may be comforting. And a thorough, honest and objective assessment of your own personality may help you ascertain its effects on the role pain plays in your life.

# 5

## DIAGNOSING PAIN

*T*here's an age-old adage every doctor learns in medical school that says, "Diagnosis is the cornerstone of treatment." And though the adage might seem almost laughingly obvious, the proper diagnosis of a patient's symptoms can prove quite the opposite. And if that's the case, then neither patient nor doctor will be laughing, for an improper diagnosis usually leads to improper treatment—which, for a chronic pain victim could prove disastrous.

Diagnosing the underlying cause of chronic pain in the typical patient is an extremely difficult task even in the best of circumstances. It can be a long, grueling process and exact a terrible toll on both patient and physician.

After all, pain is a subjective experience that can't be measured in any kind of concrete, numerical terms; consequently, objective, quantifying tests—such as asking the patient, "How much does it hurt?"—are useless.

The old standby tests such as the physical exam and nerve-conduction studies are okay as far as they go, but fail to take into account that chronic pain is a disease in itself and do not address the special, individual problems a patient may have. Standard diagnostic tools including X-rays and electromyographic studies (referring to tests of muscle power and strength) can pinpoint organic causes of pain complaints. These tests can find lesions on nerves, degenerating muscles, inflammation of joints and imbalances of body fluids, all of which cause pain. But there are a myriad of other pain syndromes, and a great number of them are obscure, unpublicized in medical literature and *much* more difficult to find than is the typical needle in that proverbial haystack.

Moreover, when the medical community decided to get serious about chronic pain, it had to develop new techniques, devices and methods to locate the source of pain in a given patient, so the person's problem could be accurately diagnosed and the proper treatment prescribed.

What follows are brief descriptions of some of the tools used by physicians over the past 10 to 15 years to diagnose chronic pain.

**EMG and NCV Studies**—Electromyographic studies (EMG) and nerve-conduction velocity studies (NCV) are used to investigate whether damage has occurred in nerves supplying muscles or in the muscles themselves as the result of compression, disc herniation, scar-tissue formation, sectioning, entrapment, or crush injury. In order to measure these changes, small needles are inserted into the muscles (in the case of EMG studies) and near nerves (in the case of NCV studies). Should there be a change in the nerve supply of a muscle or damage to the muscle itself, changes in electrical energy in the muscle are measured and recorded on a TV screen called an oscilloscope. These recordings can be photographed and computer-recorded for future recall.

While NCVs use the same technique, they actually measure the velocity with which a nerve conducts an impulse. If the speed of conduction is slow, there is proof that nerve damage has occurred.

EMG and NCV studies help localize the damage that can occur, but they do not measure pain. This is an important consideration since very often, people will have normal EMG and NCV studies, but will still experience pain. Likewise, they may have abnormal EMG and NCV studies and not experience any pain.

**Nerve Blocks**—are used when it's unclear which nerve or group of nerves is causing the patient's pain. A local anesthetic, or numbing agent, is injected around the nerve sheath (the membrane covering the nerve). If the pain disappears during the time the medicine works (usually ninety minutes to four hours), then returns when the medicine wears off, the pain source has been identified and treatment of the nerve can begin. Several injections on successive days may be required to locate the offending nerve.

**Thermography**—is a specialized test used to detect temperature differences in the body caused by cancer growth or by injuries to the nervous system or blood vessels. Infra-red, heat-sensitive detection devices measure the temperature of the top 7–10 mm. of skin, with photographs taken of the affected areas to document the thermographic images. Areas of pain show up as cool spots, while warm spots denote cancer. This test has been grossly misused and overused, but it is of great value in the early detection of reflex sympathetic dystrophy, causalgia and thoracic outlet syndrome.

**Bone Scan**—A bone scan is ordered in order to rule out the possibility of infection that may occur after an operation, or for detecting hidden fractures that might not be picked up on X-ray. Bone scans are also useful for detecting reduced blood flow in a bone, arthritic joints and/or arthritis around joints, that might escape detection on X-ray because of prostheses.

A bone scan measures the metabolic activity of the bone. It is performed by injecting a radioactive tracer into the body, allowing it to accumulate on the bone, and then scanning the entire body with X-ray. The tracer remains in the body for only a short period of time. Healing fractures, recent breaks, infections and other disorders cause increased metabolic activity in the bone. A bone scan can determine whether one of the aforementioned is taking place in the area of pain. Bone scans are especially useful when the X-rays do not show any pathology. Sometimes X-rays miss certain problems; the bone scan may help to detect them.

The radioactive tracer gallium has increased uptake in areas of the bone and in soft tissue where infection is present. If a bone scan has positive findings, but the source of the abnormality cannot be determined, the gallium scan can help differentiate the source of the problem. In other words, with a positive bone scan and a positive gallium scan, a doctor can usually determine that the source of the pain is due specifically to infection, rather than an undetected break in the bone, or an area of slow healing.

**CAT Scan**—or computed tomographic scan—is a test that uses computers, X-rays and Polaroid-type pictures to give cross-section views of all parts of the body, including the brain. A CAT scan requires the patient to lie perfectly still with his arms over his head inside an X-ray device that looks like a futuristic coffin, made of steel and attached to rotating platforms. The test lasts about 45 minutes and yields dozens of images allowing physicians to see the various cross-sections of an organ instead of just the outline or silhouette.

CAT scans are effective for detecting cysts and for locating problems in soft tissue, such as abnormalities within the liver, brain, abdomen and lung. But the best use of a CAT scan is for outlines of bony structures, detecting breaks and lesions that X-rays and even bone scans miss.

**MRI**—or magnetic resonance imaging—is a technique used to examine soft tissue with even greater accuracy than a CAT scan. In this test, a powerful magnetic force is applied to the tissue, aligning water molecules within the body and generating an image particularly useful for viewing the brain as well as the spinal area for detection of abnormal discs, scar tissue and nerve roots.

**Myelogram**—a word every patient prays never crosses his doctor's lips, a word capable of striking terror into the strongest person. Indeed, the person who coined the phrase, "the cure is worse than the disease," had probably just undergone a myelogram. Of course it's not a cure for anything, but rather a procedure that helps the doctor determine whether a pain is caused by pressure on the spinal cord or on the nerves that leave the spinal cord (nerve roots).

A myelogram uses a radio-opaque dye (one that acts as a shield against X-rays) that is injected into the spinal canal. It appears on the X-ray as a white substance contouring the discs, the sac that surrounds the spinal cord and various bony areas.

Despite recent advances in CAT scan and MRI, nothing shows up lesions within the spinal canal quite as well as a myelogram. However, the myelogram is not infallible, and can miss herniated discs that are otherwise picked up by MRI, or at the time of surgery. A myelogram is also good at detecting the presence or absence of scar tissue within the spinal canal, but again it's not infallible.

In the past, the dye used for myelograms was oil-based and thus needed to be drawn out after testing. Consequently, it was necessary to leave the needle in the patient's back throughout the test. This tended to create a leakage of fluid from the sac surrounding the spinal cord resulting in headaches for some patients.

The oil-based dye was also known to cause inflammatory reactions with some patients.

Today, a water-soluble dye, metrizamide, is used. The dye doesn't need to be drawn out and thus the needle doesn't remain in the patient's back. In addition, the chance of an inflammatory reaction from metrizamide is virtually unknown.

Unfortunately, metrizamide has its own set of side effects. In combination with certain medications (notably antidepressants and some antihistamines) the dye may precipitate seizures. Therefore, a patient should inform his doctor of all medications that he is taking prior to the metrizamide myelogram.

**3-D CAT Scan**—In 1978, the most sophisticated method for investigating spinal problems was a combination of the metrizamide myelogram and a CAT scan. The radio-opaque dye helped outline anatomical structures so they showed up better on the myelogram. They dye also enhanced the image of the CAT scan, producing a higher degree of contrast between objects inside the sac around the spinal cord and those objects outside the sac. We believed this method caught nearly one hundred percent of any abnormality that might have existed—until the three-dimensional CAT scan came into use.

For all the reasons CAT scans are effective, 3-D CAT scans are even better, because the spinal cord and vertebra may be viewed from the inside out. In addition, viewing angles can be changed, often times revealing subtle lesions that weren't visible from a single viewpoint. In fact, recent research conducted at Johns Hopkins Hospital showed how 3-D CAT scans were able to detect bony breaks missed by bone scans, regular CAT scans, X-rays, MRI and myelograms.

**Flexion Extension X-rays**—Most X-rays are mistakenly taken with the patient standing erect. These are virtually useless, especially if the patient has been subjected to a fall, hyperextension or hyperflexion or a twisting type injury. Very often patients complain of worse pain when they lean forward, or backwards, or twist to one side. Therefore, it makes no sense to take X-rays while the patient is standing still, but is better to take the X-ray while the patient is engaged in the motion that produces the pain they experience.

This type of X-ray is useful for detecting disorders such as spondylolysis, and spondylolisthesis. Spondylolysis is a break in the pars inter-articularis of the vertebral body, while spondylolisthesis is a break with displacement of the bone of the pars inter-articularis of the vertebral body. These X-rays are also useful for detecting subluxation, which is a tearing of the ligaments between the vertebral bodies whereby one vertebral body can slip either forward or backwards upon the other one, causing compression of the spinal cord and nerve roots.

**QFM**—or Quantitative flow meter, a sophisticated Doppler study available at a few pain clinics that measures not only the blood flow within a particular artery, but also the diameter of the artery itself, information needed to detect vascular occlusions and vascular components of thoracic outlet syndrome.

**Provocative Discogism**—often times a disc will not protrude into the spinal canal, thereby escaping detection by CAT scan, MRI or myelogram. But a disrupted disc doesn't have to press on the spinal cord or nerve root to cause the joint between two vertebral bodies to move more than it should. This movement is called an instability and can create pain when a person so afflicted moves back and forth.

To test for this condition, the patient is first given an injection of Versed, a substance that will keep him awake during the procedure but wipe out his memory.

Next, a radiologist inserts a needle into the disc, guided by instantaneous X-ray (called fluoroscopic control) to assure it is placed correctly. Then a small (1cc–2cc) amount of saline (salt water) is injected into the disc, and the doctor asks his patient for a verbal reaction.

Then a numbing agent (Marcain) is injected into the same spot with the same needle, and the patient is again asked how he feels.

Finally, dye is injected into the disc and a CAT scan or MRI is administered to discover whether or not it leaks out.

**Indirium III Test**—a test for infection in which blood is removed from the patient under sterile conditions and radioactive particles attached to the white blood cells. The patient returns the next day, and his blood is reinjected. The patient is then given a scan—most likely an X-ray—to search for infection. Because white blood cells travel to areas of infection in the body, and because *these* white blood cells have been subjected to ultra-low level radiation to make them appear brighter on the scan than normal tissue, any areas of infection will be readily revealed. If there is no infection present, the white blood cells will disperse evenly into the patient's blood and there will be no bright spots on the scan.

**Facet Blocks**—The facets are joints that exist between each vertebral body. This is a real joint, with its own capsule, disc and synovial fluid, as well as nervous innervation. There are three positions of the vertebral body where an anesthesiologist, orthopedic surgeon or neurosurgeon performs facet blocks. These are at the transverse process, at the pars inter-articularis or a the capsule (joint) itself. In fact, some anesthesiologists have perfected a technique of performing facet arthrogram whereby dye is injected into the facet capsules to determine whether or not this capsule is ruptured. The purpose of performing facet blocks is simple. Very often patients with back pain explain that when they lean backwards, pain shoots down the leg, but rarely below the knee. This very often is facet pain rather than root pain. A trial with facet blocks obviates the need for a myelogram or CAT scan and assists in the diagnosis of a patient. If the facet blocks are effective, then facet denervation may be accomplished, which is merely burning out the nerve that creates the problem in the first place.

## How Much Pain Do You Feel?

While any number of tests can and may be used to detect and pinpoint the presence of pain in a patient, a simple psychological screening exam will usually suffice in clarifying the non-physiological problems both patient and physician will encounter in determining a final diagnosis and method(s) of treatment.

Perhaps you have already encountered some of the tests used to analyze a variety of complaints from people, including chronic-pain patients, who seek psychiatric help. One of the most common screening tests for personality disorders or for simple personality evaluation is the Minnesota Multiphasic Personality Inventory (MMPI), which contains nearly six hundred true or false questions that a person answers himself. Another test that has gained acceptance is the SCL 90-R with ninety questions which are also answered on a score sheet.

Based on the results of the MMPI, psychiatrists and psychologists determine the personality traits of their patients. In particular, the MMPI picks out such characteristics as hysteria or a tendency to hypochondria, or it determines whether or not the patient is anxious or depressed. Some scientists and physicians use this test to predict the outcome of treatment: how well a person will respond to treatment, if he will recover (particularly pertinent in the case of a preoperative patient).

Some physicians believe, however, that the MMPI is an invalid tool for diagnosing chronic-pain patients because although it has built-in safeguards against internal inconsistencies, the test does not take into account personality factors that change over time. Filling in an answer sheet without supervision allows the patient to interpret the questions as he wishes, and this leaves room for misinterpretation of the intent of the questions. The patient may also prejudge his answer before he puts it down and decide that another response might show him in a better light, thereby skewing his score. And finally, the test is not specifically designated for pain patients.

The SCL 90-R, created by Leonard Derogatis, Ph.D., at Johns Hopkins Hospital, evaluates complaints over a period of time. This test is a list of problems and complaints ranging from headaches, faintness, or dizziness to the feeling that people are unfriendly and don't like you. The patient marks the ninety statements to indicate how much discomfort ("not at all," "a little bit," "a great deal") any particular problem has caused him over a period of time, up to and including the day of the test. This test has its limitations too, since it requires the patient to judge how he feels, subject to his own interpretation rather than to the observation of a trained clinician. However, it has the advantage of being able to assess changes in a person's feelings over time.

Some pain treatment clinics develop their own diagnostic tests, usually containing the best features of the MMPI and SCL 90-R with innovative questions devised by the staff based on the observations of former pain patients. For example, here's a ten-minute-screening test for chronic back-pain patients developed at the Johns Hopkins Chronic Pain Treatment Center in conjunction with Dr. Donlin Long, the center's director and professor of neurosurgery at the hospital.

The following Screening Test for Chronic Back Pain Patients is designed to screen patients for the purpose of facilitating appropriate treatment decisions. As a pain victim, you also will be able to see how you handle chronic pain and how pain affects you. The test should take you about ten minutes to complete. For each question circle the statement that most closely applies to you, and mark down the number of points you receive on a separate sheet of paper. This test is specifically designed for back pain and may not accurately reflect responses to other types of pain.

I    When did you first notice the pain that you now experience?
    (a)   Sudden onset after/with an accident or definable event.    0
    (b)   Slow, progressive onset, with sharp accompanying pain.    1
    (c)   Slow, progressive onset, without sharp accompanying pain.    2
    (d)   A sudden onset of pain without an accident or event to which you can tie the pain.    3

II    Where do you feel the pain?
    (a)   One specific, well-defined place.    0
    (b)   Several different places.    1
    (c)   One place, but hard to tell exactly where.    2
    (d)   It's hard to describe exactly where the pain is, and it feels different in different places. No physician has been able to tie it to a specific source.    3

III    Do you have trouble falling asleep at night?
    No. (If no, go to question V.)
    Yes. (If yes, go to question IV.)

IV    What keeps you from falling asleep at night?
    (a)   I have trouble falling asleep at night because of pain, and I'm awakened by the pain every night.    0
    (b)   Because of the pain, I have trouble falling asleep about three times a week or more, and I'm awakened by the pain from sleep more than three times a week.    1

(c)   I have trouble falling asleep more than three times a week, but I'm not awakened from sleep by the pain more than twice a week. 2

(d)   I have no trouble falling asleep because of the pain, and it does not wake me once I'm asleep.

3

(e)   I have trouble falling asleep, or I'm awakened early in the morning—but it's not because of the pain.                                    4

V   Does the weather have any effect on your pain?

(a)   The pain is always worse with *both* cold and damp weather.                                    0

(b)   The pain is always worse with *either* cold or damp weather.                                    1

(c)   The pain is occasionally worse with cold or damp weather.                                    2

(d)   The weather has no effect on the pain.    3

VI   How would you describe the type of pain you have now?

(a)   Burning, or sharp, shooting pain, or pins and needles, or coldness, or numbness.        0

(b)   Dull, aching pain, with occasional sharp shooting pains, not helped by heat applications; or sense of cold or heat to touch.            1

(c)   Spasm-type pain, tension-type pain, or a numbness over the area of pain helped by massage and heat.                                    2

(d)   Nagging or bothersome pain.            3

(e)   Excruciating, overwhelming, or unbearable pain, relieved by heat or massage.        4

VII   How frequently do you have pain?

(a)   The pain is constant.                        0

(b) The pain is nearly constant, fifty to eighty
percent of the time.                                    1

(c) The pain is intermittent, twenty-five to fifty
percent of the time.                                    2

(d) The pain is only occasionally present, less than
twenty-five percent of the time.                        3

VIII Does movement of position have any effect on the
pain?

(a) The pain is unrelieved by a position change or
when I don't use that part of my body where
it hurts. I also have a history of previous
operations for the pain.                                0

(b) The pain gets worse when I use that part of my
body where it hurts or when I stand or walk.
It's relieved when I lie down, or when I don't
use that part of my body where it hurts.        1

(c) The pain is affected according to my position
or my use of the part of my body where it hurts.
2

(d) There is no change in the pain with a change
in position or use of the part of my body where
it hurts. I have not had any operations for the
pain.                                                   3

IX What medications have you used in the past month?

(a) No medication at all.                               0

(b) I've used a non-narcotic pain reliever or a mild
tranquilizer (non-benzodiazepam) or an anti
depressant.                                             1

(c) I've used a strong painkiller or a sleeping pill
less than three times a week, or I've taken a
(benzodiazepam) tranquilizer less than three
times a week.                                           2

(d) I've used either a painkiller or a sleeping pill or a tranquilizer (benzodiazepam) more than four times a week. 3

X What hobbies do you have? Can you still participate in them?

(a) I am unable to participate at all in any hobbies I used to enjoy. 0

(b) I've reduced my number of hobbies or activities relating to the hobbies. 1

(c) I still participate in my hobbies, but with some discomfort. 2

(d) I participate in my hobbies the same as before. 3

XI How frequently did you have sex and orgasms before the pain? How frequently do you have sex and orgasms now?

(a) I had a good sexual relationship prior to the pain, about three or four times a week, with no difficulty with orgasm, but now I have sexual contacts less than once a week and that is interrupted by the pain. 0

(b) Before the pain, I had a good sexual relationship, about three or four times a week, with no difficulty with orgasms, but now I have less interest in sex, have sex less than once a week, and have difficulty with orgasm or erection. 1

(c) There has been no change in my sexual activity. It is the same now as it was before I began experiencing the pain. 2

(d) I am unable to have any sexual contact since the pain, and I had difficulty with orgasms or erection prior to the pain. 3

XII  Are you still working or doing your household chores?

    (a)  I work every day at the same job I had prior to the onset of my pain, at the same level and with the same duties.     0

    (b)  I work every day, but the job is not the same as I had before the onset of pain. I have reduced responsibilities or fewer activities.     1

    (c)  I work sporadically, or I have reduced my household chores.     2

    (d)  I don't work any more, someone else does my household chores.     3

XIII  What is your income now compared to the time before your injury or the beginning of your pain? What are the sources of your income?

    (a)  I'm experiencing financial difficulty, and my family income has been cut in half or more since the onset of pain.     0

    (b)  I'm experiencing some financial difficulty, with my family income fifty to seventy percent of the pre-pain income.     1

    (c)  I am unable to work; I receive some compensation and my spouse works, so my income is at least seventy-five percent of my pre-pain income.     2

    (d)  My income is about eighty percent or more of my gross pay before the pain, and my spouse does not work.     3

XIV  Are you suing anyone, or is anyone suing you, or do you have an attorney helping you with compensation or disability payment?

    (a)  I have no suits pending, and I do not have an attorney.     0

   (b)   I have a suit pending, but it is not related to the pain.    1

   (c)   I am being sued as the result of an accident.    2

   (d)   I have a suit pending, or I am expecting workmen's compensation, and I have a lawyer involved.    3

XV  If you had three wishes for anything in the world, what would you wish for?

   (a)   "Get rid of the pain" is the only wish I would have for all three wishes.    0

   (b)   "Get rid of the pain" would be one of my three wishes.    1

   (c)   My wishes would be something of a personal nature, such as having more money, having a better relationship with my spouse or my children, and having a bigger house.    2

   (d)   My wishes would be for something like peace in the world, an end to hunger, or something else for others.    3

XVI  Have you ever been depressed or thought of suicide?

   (a)   I have been depressed, or I have been depressed in addition to having pain. My depression makes me cry at times or think of suicide.    0

   (b)   Because of pain, I've been depressed, and I've felt guilty and angry.    1

   (c)   I felt depressed before the pain, or before the pain I suffered a financial or personal loss (death of a friend, family member moved away), and now with the pain here, I also have some depression.    2

(d)  I don't feel depressed, I don't have crying jags, or I don't feel blue.                    3

(e)  Before the pain I had a history of suicide attempts.                    4

*Add up all your points.* A score of 17 points or less suggests that you are a Type I personality (a coper) and are showing the normal response to chronic pain. You are usually willing to participate in suggested therapy, including exercise and supportive psychotherapy.

Based on recent research, there is a 94% chance you have a physical problem that would be identified by at least one objective test.

A score of 18–20 points indicates that you exhibit features of both a coper and an exaggerator. Therefore, there's a 75% chance that you have an organic problem that will show up on laboratory testing, but you may also have had some problems that pre-existed or were unrelated to the pain.

A score of 21–31 points suggest that you are a Type II personality (the exaggerator). Surgical or other intervention procedures may be recommended for you with caution. The test shows that you may have found a use for chronic pain. You may benefit from treatment at a chronic-pain center with an emphasis on attitude change toward the chronic pain.

A score of 32 points or more suggests that a psychiatric consultation is needed. You are the type of personality that freely admits that you had a great many pre-pain problems and that you have a great deal of difficulty coping with the chronic pain you now have. Surgical or other intervention procedures should not be carried out without prior approval of a psychiatric consultant.

(Copyright 1977, Nelson Hendler, M.D. This questionnaire or portions of this questionnaire may not be duplicated, printed or copied without the express written permission of the author.)

# 6

## THERAPIES AND TREATMENTS
## TO HELP YOU COPE

*O*nce the source of pain has been located and identified, the patient and his doctor must decide upon a program of therapy they believe will be most effective in achieving relief.

Just as there are a number of tests that may or may not be of use during the diagnostic stage, chronic-pain therapy may involve a host of treatment procedures, singly or in combination, for any amount of time, from two weeks to several months to many years.

On the following pages we list and briefly examine some of the most widely used and readily available methods for the treatment of chronic pain.

A number of these treatments may be offered at the private offices of some physical therapists or physicians and at some general hospitals. However, they can be found in the greatest concentration at pain clinics.

Some pain clinics treat only specific kinds of pain or a particular form of therapy. For example, there are clinics devoted exclusively to the treatment of head-aches or backaches. There are some clinics that use only anesthetics and others that use only nerve blocks in their therapy. However, it is the multi-disciplinary pain clinic, where a variety of treatments are available, that seems to have the best record in relief offered and obtained.

## Drug Withdrawal

Pain-clinic physicians often request that new patients bring in all the prescription and over-the-counter drugs they are taking at the time of their admission or have taken in the past for their pain. Some patients literally bring in a shopping bag filled with pills and admit to taking all of them. Some of the medications may be harmless. Some may be placebos—sugar pills pre-scribed by a physician who didn't believe "the pain was real" but wanted to give his patient something to assuage his fears.

Some pills are harmful; they can be addicting, depressing or they might even worsen the pain. Some pills, for example, when taken in combination with others, can potentiate the intended effect of both drugs and lead to mood changes, body-chemistry changes, coma or death from overdose.

Unfortunately, the most widely prescribed drugs for chronic pain are addicting. Addiction occurs when your body reaches a tolerance level for a prescribed dosage of a drug and then requires a larger dose for it to have the same effect it once had. As you increase your tolerance level, you must ingest more and more of the drug until at last you can't function during the day without it—your body chemistry has been altered and needs it to feel "normal" or "well."

If you are addicted to painkillers, sleeping pills or tranquilizers, they have probably become part of your daily routine, and you swallow them without thinking. But they might also be contributing to your pain either through a direct effect on your body (where the drugs themselves are causing pain or discomfort) or an incidental side effect (such as when the drugs induce drowsiness, keeping you in bed all day when what your body actually needs is physical exercise to help rid itself of the pain). The benzodiazepines (Valium, Librium, et al.) are a case in point. They are prescribed by well-intentioned doctors to their patients who complain of chronic pain, but in fact may worsen pain.

A vicious circle begins with the first prescription. Benzodiazepines may alleviate anxiety for a time, but never to the root of pain. So when the pain returns, the patient takes more pills, until he or she reaches the point where he takes the pills before the pain comes, because his body requires them.

Barbiturate sleeping pills (such as Seconal or Tuinal) are also frequently prescribed, easily abused and addictive. They are prescribed when the patient complains that either he can't get to sleep at night because of the pain or that he has trouble staying asleep. Again the doctor means well, but all he's really doing is contributing to the pain-pill cycle. Frequently patients who are "on" sleeping pills need amphetamines to wake them up in the morning, and then they need the sleeping pills at night to counter the effects of the stimulants.

By the time a chronic-pain patient has accumulated a shopping bag of pills, his life is built around his medication. When he arrives at the pain clinic, the staff will assess his drugs. They need to see how the patient functions and feels without the pills, so withdrawal is initiated. They need to see his reaction to the pain without the dulling effect of drugs.

For some people withdrawal from drugs may be quite simple. The staff takes away the pills and does not provide any more unless a staff physician orders them. Period. The patient is withdrawn.

For others drug withdrawal may be a slow, gradual process. The body must get accustomed once again to functioning without the pills. Usually the body cannot stand the shock of instant withdrawal (cold turkey). So the treatment center doles the drugs out in increasingly smaller doses until the body can handle not having any drugs at all.

Drug withdrawal is not offered as a sole treatment in a pain clinic. It is an adjunctive therapy. It works best when undertaken voluntarily and with a total commitment.

## Prescribing Drugs

Although pain clinics usually advocate withdrawal from all drugs, treatment may consist of a pharmaceutical regimen. How drugs work and why they are used will be discussed thoroughly in a later chapter.

## Surgery

Surgery is the most complex and serious treatment recommended by pain clinics and should be avoided if a different method of treatment is available and effective. However, in some cases surgery is a chronic-pain patient's only hope for relief.

For example, people with trigeminal neuralgia, or tic douloureux, are often treated with anticonvulsive drugs such as Dilantin or Tegretol that control the agony for a time, but surgery is usually called for eventually.

One of the newest procedures developed to aid the victims of this dreaded disorder is percutaneous rhizotomy (an operation that is, in part, performed on an awake and alert patient). The surgeon guides a needle-thin electrode through the patient's cheek to the appropriate offending nerve. During this procedure the patient is awake so he can tell the surgeon whether he has found the correct nerve. The surgeon then thermocoagulates the nerve (heats the nerve until the pain fibers are destroyed), effectively cutting off the energy supply to the cheek. The thermocoagulation portion of the surgery is performed with the patient under general anesthesia.

As with any operation there are drawbacks because of the potential side effects of the procedure. In this particular operation there is the possibility that the patient will have anesthesia of his face in the area of the surgery (meaning that the face will feel numb). Another possible side effect is a weakening of the chewing muscles on the operated side. (Of course, the patient would be advised of such surgical side effects prior to the operation. It is up to him to weigh the benefits and risks with the help of his physician before deciding to undergo the procedure. Most tic douloureux victims are willing to exchange their pain for muscle numbness or weakness.)

A surgical procedure for chronic-pain patients suffering from back pain is a disc operation. Diseased discs either can be fixed, partially removed, or fully removed. In many cases these procedures reduce or totally alleviate the pain.

## Nerve Blocks

If the offending agent in the life of the chronic-pain patient is an injured nerve, a block of this nerve may be recommended by the pain-clinic staff. Nerve blocks are procedures during which an anesthesiologist injects a local anesthetic into a nerve to cut off its function. If its energy is cut, the nerve message is interrupted and does not reach the brain.

As noted in Chapter 5, nerve blocks also can be used as a diagnostic tool. If the staff is unsure which nerve or group of nerves is causing the patient's pain, an anesthesiologist may be called in. On successive days, he will block different nerves with an anesthetic, until both he and the patient are certain of the locations. Further treatment at this point may be either to continue blocking the offending nerve or to perform surgery—an incision or excision of the nerve so that its energy source is permanently cut off.

## Electrical Stimulators

Electrical stimulators are devices used by pain clinics and physical therapists and by some private physicians to help combat pain by interrupting pain-nerve messages. Some of these devices are transcutaneous (across the skin) and some are implanted under the skin. At one pain clinic the devices have been successful with about forty percent of the patients who have tried them, but success depends on the type of pain.

The transcutaneous electrical stimulator merely applies a low-voltage current between two electrodes on the skin. The stimulator is composed of a radio transmitter (a small plastic circle that sends impulses through the skin to a receiver that is taped to the lower back) and a power pack. The transmitter sends impulses to the receiver; the impulses block incoming pain messages traveling along the spinal cord. The power pack (which is about the size and shape of a cigarette pack and can be tucked away in a shirt pocket) sends electrical impulses to the transmitter. Patients who have used this device successfully say they feel a pleasant, warm, tingling sensation. Others find the stimulator's sensation irritating.

Electrical stimulators are also designed so that the receiver component can be implanted in the back or even in the brain, where the effect is thought to be more potent.

In some pain clinics, the stimulator, a prescription item, is used as adjunctive therapy, rather than as a single treatment. If it proves effective, it may be continuously worn by the patient, even when he sleeps.

## Psychotherapy

Individual psychotherapy may offer support or employ supportive measures, or it may seek to find the source of problems using a variety of techniques. These therapies help both the professional and the patient to explore the patient's personality and behavior patterns to determine how chronic pain fits into his life and to define and measure his emotional needs. Psychotherapy also seeks to help the patient find solutions to his problem by revealing his personality traits and guiding him toward insights about his flaws and strengths.

## Group Therapy

Group therapy is a treatment utilizing the dynamics of group interaction to achieve therapy and treatment for the individual patients in the group.

What are group dynamics? They include the reaction of individuals to one another in a group, role playing by the individual group members, the assumption of the leadership role by someone in the group and how this occurs, how followers react to the leader, and how each individual responds to the questions or statements of the other members of the group.

Individual members of groups learn from one another by seeing how they look and sound to other people. A group leader can be designated to act as a "facilitator of group dynamics." The group leader may be a psychiatrist, a licensed therapist, a social worker or a member of the group.

In a pain clinic, group therapy deals with not only the responses and actions of individuals while they are in session together (usually for an hour each day), but it also includes all the interactions among patients on the ward. In pain clinics, chronic-pain patients eat together, take the recommended exercise therapy together, make their own beds, visit the nurses' station together to receive their medication, and talk to one another when-

ever they meet on the ward. They are continually inter-
acting with one another, testing their behavior on these
intimate strangers who in some ways share their pain. A
camaraderie develops among the patients and with it an
understanding of how their fellow patients suffer. All
this communication and interaction is therapy that helps
chronic-pain patients readjust their thinking. They see
what being ill and acting ill does to each of them and how
other people cope with pain. They learn that their
method of handling pain is not the only way, and that
they're not the only people in the world who suffer from
pain. This realization alone is therapeutic.

In an actual group session there are from five to
fifteen people who participate in the discussion. If there
are fewer than five, significant group dynamics won't
take place; the group is too small for effective interaction
to occur. And with more than fifteen people, the group
is too large for effective action; some members will be
lost in the crowd.

Theoretically, groups are considered to be either
*heterogeneous*, made up of different types of members
with basically different goals for therapy (such as a group
of people waiting at a corner for a bus), or *homoge-*
*neous*, meaning the members all have a common purpose (such as a group of conventioneers waiting on a
corner for a chartered bus to take them to a lecture hall
for a continuing medical education session). Depending
on whether the group is heterogeneous or homogeneous, group dynamics will occur at different rates and
can be detrimental or beneficial to the individuals in the
group.

Sometimes no significant dynamics occur, particularly in a heterogeneous group. The group of people who meet for therapy in a pain clinic is homogeneous; the patients have similar goals (relief of pain), and their interactions tend to be beneficial. They encourage one another when good behavior is displayed and criticize those members who are acting inappropriately and possibly contributing to the continuation of their pain. How does this happen?

In the group setting, an individual is more likely to air inner feelings that he may be too embarrassed to reveal on a one-to-one basis with a therapist. The group provides a support structure. The group also allows its members to see themselves as pain patients as they look at and listen to others with pain complaints similar to their own. By comparing his behavior to others, a chronic-pain patient can see how he might help himself improve or recover.

In addition, group therapy is a useful diagnostic tool for some therapists. The interactions within a group sometimes will cause its members to physically arrange themselves into two groups: the copers—who freely admit to depression, anxiety, and other problems that their pain is causing them—on one side; the exaggerators—who refuse to admit to any of these problems, though depression or anxiety may be obvious from their outward appearance—on the other side.

The therapist might also be able to pinpoint exaggerators in a group therapy session by the way they talk about themselves. Exaggerators have a tendency to dwell on the severity of their symptoms and the degree of their incapacitation, and they try to compete with one another as to who has a greater amount of pain. Knowing which patient is a coper and which is an exaggerator helps the pain-clinic staff devise more effective treatment regimens.

Some deep-seated feelings are often brought out during a pain-clinic group-therapy session—particularly feelings of hopelessness, helplessness and worthlessness. Patients feel a degree of security in a group and are able to express these feelings in the presence of others who can respond with empathy—something that few people will do for them in their everyday lives outside the clinic setting.

Finally, group sessions help patients ventilate their anger, an emotion that can contribute to tension. The anger may be directed at the doctors who fail them, who didn't believe in their pain, or it may be directed at a family member who has forsaken them. Chronic-pain patients also bottle up anger against people they perceive as controlling their lives, people on whom they are dependent and to whom they are now obligated. They may also be angry at themselves for having gotten into the position of being dependent, or for somehow having brought the pain on themselves. Ventilating anger also is therapeutic; it can release tension and is also a part of the attitude change that pain clinics seek.

## Family Therapy

Family therapy emerged in the mid-1950s when psychiatrists and psychologists decided to examine a phenomenon they saw occurring in some of the relatives of their patients. It seems as a patient improves, his relatives, rather than acting grateful or relieved, were suspicious and almost unhappy with the improvement. The families sought to pull the patient out of treatment or in some other way to subtly undermine the benefits the therapist was achieving. A good example of this phenomenon is the adolescent who, having achieved some success on a diet prescribed by her physician and vocally urged on by her mother, is suddenly told by that same mother that she is too thin and should start eating more—even though the girl has not yet reached her weight goal.

As in groups, there is a system of dynamics or interaction that occurs within families. Each person in the family has a role and the power that goes with the role. Members of families interact with one another by wielding that power, mostly to maintain their position in the family.

Thus psychiatrists and their colleagues have surmised that if one member of a family is emotionally or mentally ill, the illness probably has had an effect on other members of the family, too. Therefore, it would not be productive to treat the person with the problem without also treating the relatives who will be instrumental in either helping him recover or prolonging his illness. In other words, not only is the patient sick but his family may be sick as well, and in order for the patient to regain his health, the family unit must also regain its health.

For example, if an adult, an exaggerator-type pain patient, has to move back in with his mother to receive the kind of care he needs, his mother may enjoy assuming the role of "mother" again—after having relinquished it when her child grew up and moved out of the house to be on his own. The mother might undermine the effects of therapy by keeping her child in bed, providing for his every whim, even though the therapist has suggested that the patient move around as much as possible and stay out of bed until it's time to go to sleep.

A family therapist would call the mother into therapy with her son to discuss why she is keeping her son in bed, to help her explore her motives, and to show her why it is necessary that her son move about the house. Once the mother understands that her efforts to keep him dependent and at home are detrimental to his health, she can perhaps learn to let go and thereby help her son on the road to recovery.

## Occupational Therapy

Occupational therapy aims to provide patients with marketable skills to compensate for abilities their pain has taken from them. If a warehouseman experiences chronic pain because he was injured lifting a heavy load the wrong way, the occupational therapist can teach him the proper way to lift lighter loads or train him for an entirely different job—one he can use without having to change employers; for instance, he might learn to be an inventory clerk.

This type of therapy can be extremely helpful in providing the patient with both economic and emotional stability. Not only will the patient's new skills give him an opportunity to keep earning money without having to look elsewhere for work, they also should reduce his anxiety and give him something to focus on apart from his current incapacity. He maintains confidence in his ability to be productive and conquer pain.

## Behavior Modification

Behavior modification is a way of changing behavior (what you do) with a system of rewards for good behavior, to encourage it to continue, and another system of punishments for bad behavior, to discourage its repetition. The cause for the action is not examined—only the action itself. Behavior modification for chronic-pain patients will be discussed more thoroughly in Chapter 8.

## Biofeedback

Biofeedback was once considered a counterculture fad, a part of the meditation movement that promised to bring its advocates nirvana or inner peace by helping them achieve their "alpha state," a restful state somewhere between consciousness and sleep.

But now the focus has moved away from alpha brain waves, and medical investigators have adapted biofeedback as a mechanism for teaching people a new awareness of their bodies and the way it works as a means of achieving something more tangible than inner peace—that being relaxation and/or health. For example, by using the biofeedback machine you can become aware that a particular event, mood, thought or person makes you tense (and tension, as you know, contributes to spasms and pain), and then you can learn to avoid it.

Biofeedback machines resemble a stack of stereo components—complete with knobs, swaying needles and dials—and measure energy output from muscles and body temperature. The electromyographic biofeedback machine, with the use of a computer and electrodes attached to specific muscles or critical temperature or pulse points, can teach the user to control certain physiological processes. The user can see what is going on in his body and how it is reacting by looking at either an instantaneous display, a graphic representation or an average activity over a period of time, depending on the model for machine in use.

Biofeedback has been found useful in reducing pain caused by spasms, migraine headaches and tension. But exactly how it works is a matter of debate.

Some experts suggest biofeedback gives the patient a sense of control over his pain; others say the process distracts his attention from the pain to the process itself. There are those who believe biofeedback produces a hypnotic-like suggestion in the user, and others think it serves as a teaching mechanism, that by showing a person on a graph or ticker tape how different actions affect his pain, he can learn to manipulate the pain by manipulating the graph.

For example, if the biofeedback's electrodes are placed on his temples and he clenches his jaws, he actually will see a rise in the tension of his muscles, graphically represented by a meter.

Therefore, if electrodes are attached to the point where a low-back-pain patient feels pain and he watches that pain (as muscle tension) register on the graph, he should be able to reduce his discomfort—if it is caused by tension—by making a conscious effort to relax. While watching the biofeedback display screen, he can try various methods of relaxing until he sees the meter reading drop. This drop should correspond to a reduction in pain.

Some researchers say this reduction in pain may be due more to a "mental calm" than a reduction in muscle spasm. This muscle calm, they suggest, comes from the feeling that he has mastered his environment, or more important, that he has come to know and master his body and its responses.

Indeed, victims of chronic pain often feel as if they have been robbed, both of good health and freedom from pain. They also feel as if they are no longer in control of their lives, creating more discomfort. Biofeedback machines teach them to take control again and in that process help them help themselves to reduce their pain.

By the way, you can purchase your own biofeedback machine and teach yourself to relax at home. For details on what to buy and how to use it, consult your physician.

## Hypnosis

Hypnosis is similar to biofeedback in that it, too, functions primarily as a tool to help the patient focus his attention away from his pain or his symptoms of pain.

It is essentially an altered state of awareness, one in which the patient is able to disassociate himself from his environment, either at the suggestion of the hypnotist or at the patient's own suggestion (autohypnosis), and concentrate on subjects or perceptions that need to be altered. The ability to concentrate this deeply varies among individuals, and not everyone *can* be hypnotized. Researchers have found that good subjects for hypnosis usually include people who are open to the suggestion that there *are* several different states of consciousness and people who take naps during the day or who are able to fall asleep whenever they want.

A pain patient undergoing hypnosis receives a suggestion from the hypnotist to imagine that he is performing some other activity; for example, he is told that instead of sitting in the hypnotist's chair, he is taking a train ride through some pretty countryside. Though the patient's central nervous system may be receiving pain messages, his perception and reception of the messages are diverted. Because of the hypnotic suggestion, the patient is absorbed in the mental image of his pleasant train ride; he feels the rhythm of the train swaying against his body—at least he imagines that he does. This enjoyable experience suppresses the pain perception, as the train ride takes center stage in the patient's state of consciousness.

The hypnotist also can plant painkilling suggestions in patients who are unable to achieve the trance-like state required to push aside all perception of pain. Some researchers have found that these posthypnotic suggestions may help make the pain tolerable. Other researchers believe hypnosis merely creates a relaxed and trusting atmosphere between patient and therapist, which helps the patient reduce his anxiety, tension and some of his pain. It also helps the patient think about his pain in a new way—to realize that pain exists only if it is perceived. If the patient can learn to modify or divert his perceptions, the impact of pain will be altered even though the stimulus that produces it still endures.

Again, as with biofeedback, you can be taught how to use hypnosis to your advantage, to achieve a peaceful and/or relaxed state that counteracts pain. But such results are temporary, and the use of hypnosis in treating chronic pain is limited.

## Acupuncture

Acupuncture was once scoffed at by Western scientists as a primitive Eastern folk remedy, on a par with a medicine man shaking a rattle to ward off evil spirits. However, just as the medicine man's techniques are now better understood by mental health professionals, so is acupuncture now seen to be of benefit in a variety of cases.

The acupuncturist uses a body chart of trigger points and a series of needles that are twisted and twirled in a certain manner at certain trigger points depending on the disease being treated and the location of the patient's chronic pain. Some needles are left in the trigger points over a period of time, twirled anywhere from ten to twenty minutes before being removed.

Scientists speculate that acupuncture may work on some patients by stimulating certain nerve pathways to send messages to the brain that counteract pain messages. It may also relieve pain caused by poor circulation by improving circulation in those areas.

Acupuncture may also achieve a placebo effect in a patient; in other words, if that patient believes the technique will help him, it *will* help him. Most significantly, however, recent research has shown acupuncture to relieve pain in a solid, concrete way by stimulating the production of a morphine-like chemical in the body.

## Heat and Massage

Two types of heat, dry and moist, will temporarily ease muscle spasm and achiness when applied directly to the body.

An easy and economical form of dry-heat therapy is a heating pad, available at most drug stores. A heat pad should be used at a medium or low setting—never on "high." It's not uncommon for patients with chronic pain to use the pad throughout the night only to awaken with first-degree burns in the morning.

The best kind of pads are those with safety-release switches. You must hold onto the switch in order for the pad to work. Obviously, when a person falls asleep, his grip on the switch relaxes, thereby shutting off the pad.

For moist heat, only use a pad designed to produce moist heat. *Do not improvise.* For example, do not wrap a wet towel around a dry-heat pad—you may run the risk of electrical shock.

One particular kind of moist heat pad is made of a rubber mat and a tube. The tube winds back and forth across the mat, similar to a refrigeration unit. A pump heats and continuously circulates warm water through the tube. This is the safest kind of heating pad, but compared to the others, it's expensive.

Hydroculator pads may provide the most professional form of moist heat. These should be used only under supervision of a physical therapist, nurse or physician. A canvas pad is filled with a gel-like substance which retains heat for a long period of time. The use of these pads, however, without proper wrapping (towels or pad covers) does present the possibility of first-degree burns.

There are various modalities of massage, ranging from applied pressure to vigorous kneading of the skin. A patient may experience increased pain during the time of the massage. This should not be a concern. However, if pain increases and persists several hours after massage, the patient can assume that massage is not an effective method of reducing pain and/or it was not applied correctly.

## Body Jacket

Body jackets can be helpful to back-pain patients who complain that their pain worsens when they lean back and/or forth. A Boston jacket is made of molded plastic and wraps around a patient to hold his spine firmly in place. This jacket is quite useful for slightly- and medium-built patients, but the heavy or overweight person should instead try a Raney flexion jacket, which has a concave vertical portion that pushes the patient's gut against the forward portion of the spinal cord for additional stability.

These jackets may also be employed during the diagnostic process, to determine the potential benefit of lumbar fusions. If a patient obtains relief from the jackets, then a fusion of the affected area will likely be successful. Indeed, it would be imprudent to perform such a fusion without first undergoing trial in a stabilizing jacket.

If both the Boston and Raney jackets prove ineffective, a trial with a body jacket with an extension around one leg provides an even more reliable test to determine the stability or instability of a particular spinal segment.

## Physical Therapy

Physical therapy is an important element of treatment because most chronic-pain patients tend to avoid any activity in order not to aggravate a painful spot. However, muscles that are not used get stiff and can cause additional pain when the patient finally attempts to use them again. For these people, walking alone may be good therapy and pain patients who undergo surgery need physical therapy following their operation to regain the use of their limbs.

For some patients, the physical therapy in pain clinics is simple and relaxing. It can take place in a small room with just one person and the therapist, or it can be a group activity set to music.

The therapy may consist of stretching motions to limber unused tendons and muscles. These movements include raising an arm up and down or moving the neck from side to side. The therapy can also include bending motions that use more than one set of muscles, such as bending from the waist with the hands dangling to the toes, then straightening the torso and bending backwards.

Because physical therapy is something you can do at home to help yourself cope with pain, we are including a list of exercises that, when done on a daily basis, constitute a useful program for most pain patients. The exercises help strengthen and stretch muscles throughout the body.

A warning: it is common to experience some muscle guarding (limitation of use) or spasms in the area of pain. This is the body's natural reaction to pain. You feel pain and you want to avoid it, so you protect yourself by not moving your muscles. This limitation of motion leads to a decreased ability to move at will and this leads to more pain. Therefore it is necessary to keep joints moving freely to help decrease muscle guarding.

———————————————

*The following are some exercises used at a major teaching hospital's pain treatment center. Check with your own physician prior to utilizing any of them. They are used primarily for back pain.*

———————————————

## Exercises
### *Easy*

STANDING:

Upper Extremities:    Ten times each
(1)   Stretch arms straight overhead, one at a time.
(2)   Stretch arms straight forward, one at a time.
(3)   Shrug shoulders, hold a few seconds, relax.
(4)   Raise arms to shoulder level, elbows bent; bring elbows backward, squeezing shoulder blades together; then stretch arms across front of body.
(5)   Do "swimming" strokes, making big circles with arms first forward, then backward.

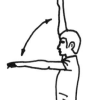

Trunk Muscles:       Ten times each
(1)   Stand with feet slightly apart; bend from waist to right side, then to left side. (Do not bend forward.)
(2)   Keep hips and lower extremities facing forward; rotate upper trunk to right; then to left.

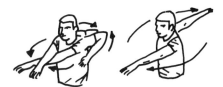

123

Lower Extremities:    Ten times each
(1)    Put one leg forward, keeping heels on floor; bend front knee (should feel stretching in back calf muscle).
(2)    March in place (at least two minutes).

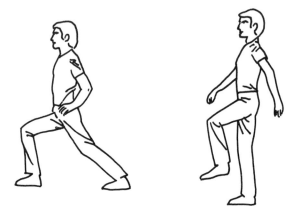

Sitting:

Lower Extremities:    Ten times each
(1)    Pull one knee up toward chest, then straighten leg; hold, and relax.
(2)    Slide to edge of chair; pull both knees up toward chest, hold, and relax (Do not lean on back of chair).
(3)    Sitting on edge of chair, bend forward bringing arms through knees to touch floor.
(4)    Lift both feet off floor; make circles with ankles.

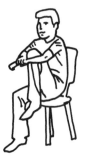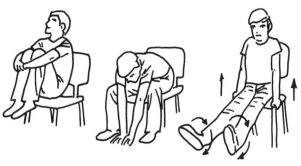

Neck Exercises:     Ten times each
(1)    Clasp hands in back of head, push head back into hands (isometric contraction), hold, and relax.
(2)    Touch chin to chest and roll shoulders forward, hold, and relax (feel stretching in back of neck).
(3)    Look straight ahead; bend head toward shoulder to right, then left. (Do not bring shoulder toward ear).
(4)    Turn head clockwise, then counterclockwise, hold, and relax.

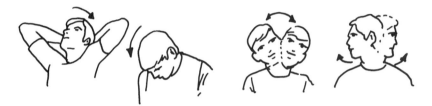

FOR THOSE WHO CAN SIT ON FLOOR:  Five times

Sit in long sitting position, legs out in front with knees straight; bend trunk forward and try to touch toes with hands.

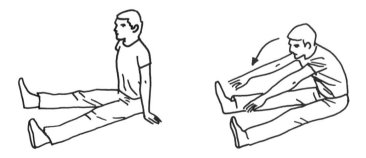

## *Advanced*

Here are some more difficult exercises. They can be used as part of a prevention program or as a way out of pain. Weak backs and unexercised muscles are vulnerable to pain. These exercises will strengthen the muscles and keep the body limber.

1. *Pelvic tilt*
a.   Begin by lying on your back with knees bent.
b.   Tighten stomach muscles and flatten lower back against floor or table, thus tipping pelvis backward; hold to count of three and relax.
c.   Repeat twenty times.

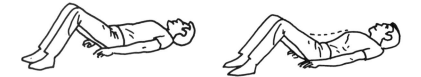

2. *Knees to chest*
a.   Begin by lying on your back with knees bent.
b.   Bend one knee toward shoulder as far as possible and return to original position.
c.   Alternate legs.
d.   Repeat ten times. Do two sets.

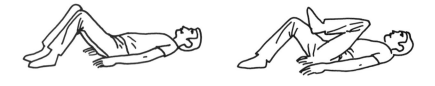

3.   *Modified bicycle*

a.   Begin by lying on your back with knees bent.

b.   Bend one knee toward chest, then straighten knee as far as possible and lower, keeping knee straight. *Keep opposite knee bent.*

c.   Alternate legs.

d.   Repeat ten times. Do two sets.

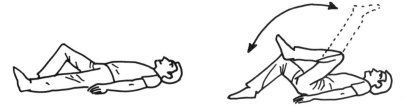

4.   *Sit-ups*

a.   Begin by lying on your back with knees bent and feet hooked under a heavy object.

b.   Hold arms straight ahead about 20 inches off the floor.

c.   Keeping arms straight, roll chin to chest and sit up as far as possible; try to roll into a ball.

d.   Return to original position slowly, keeping chin to chest.

e.   Repeat ten times. Do two sets.

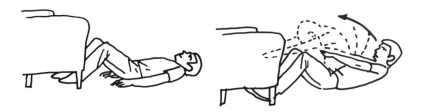

5.  *Cat's back*
a.  Begin on hands and knees
b.  Arch upper back like a cat.
c.  Bend one knee to chest; then kick the leg back, keeping knee straight and leg parallel to floor; bend knee to chest again and return to original position.
d.  Alternate legs.
e.  Repeat ten times with each leg. Do two sets.

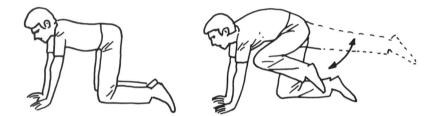

6.  *Kneel and stretch*
a.  Begin on hands and knees.
b.  Then sit back so that buttocks are resting on heels.
c.  Reach arms forward as far as possible with forehead resting on floor; keep buttocks on heels.
d.  Repeat ten times. Do two sets.

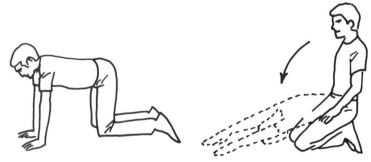

7. *Bridging*
a. Begin by lying on your back with knees bent.
b. Lift hips and buttocks off floor.
c. Hold.
d. Return to starting position.
e. Repeat ten times.

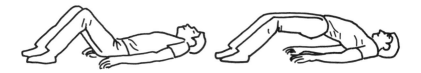

8. *Bobbing*
a. Sit on the edge of a chair that is braced against a wall.
b. Fold forearms across chest with hands hooked in the crooks of elbows.
c. Place feet flat on floor with knees well apart.
d. Put head down; drop elbows as far between legs as possible.
e. Bob toward floor five times, sit up, and repeat five times.
f. Do not drag arms down front of legs.

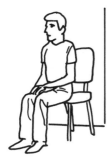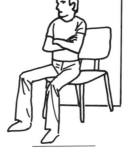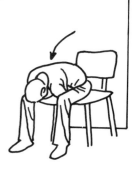

### TAKING CARE OF YOUR BACK

When standing for long periods of time, put one foot up on footstool.

Sleep best on side with both knees bent, or on back with two pillows under the knees. Avoid sleeping on the stomach.

Do not maintain any one position for any length of time; keep moving, but not necessarily vigorously.

When sitting, keep whole back supported, especially when driving.

It may help to have a small pillow in the small of the back.

Do not lift any objects weighing over three pounds. Do necessary lifting with the *legs*; bend knees to reach the floor, not waist.

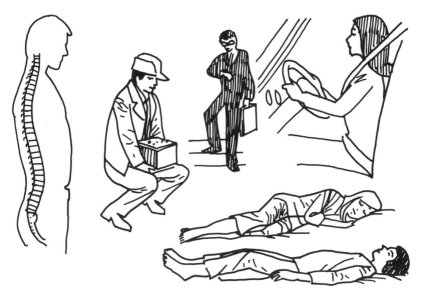

# 7

## PAIN CLINICS AND WHAT THEY CAN DO FOR YOU

*N*o *one* of the therapies we have discussed (most are available in a physician's office or hospital medical center) may be the best approach to chronic pain; however, a combination of therapies has been found to be useful in a number of cases. This kind of varied approach is offered at the multi-disciplinary pain treatment center. Multi-disciplinary means that many specialists are on hand and many more are available for consultation for each chronic-pain patient. In this era of specialists, who sometimes treat diseases just of the hand or the foot or a single organ, the multi-disciplinary team assures that the whole person will be treated.

The multi-disciplinary team that staffs a pain treatment center can be composed of a neurologist, a neurosurgeon, an orthopedic surgeon, a psychiatrist, a dentist, a radiologist, an ophthalmologist, an otolaryngologist, a pharmacologist, a social worker, a psychiatric nurse, a psychologist, a physical therapist, an internist, an occupational therapist and maybe even a scientist working on a research grant. One pain clinic in New York has nineteen different specialists available for consultation.

A pain clinic associated with a hospital can usually consult with the medical staff of the hospital if the regular staff of the clinic is baffled by a particular pain problem or patient.

The multi-disciplinary staff works together as a team, a concept of medical care especially successful with chronic-pain patients who not only present complex physical problems—but who may also suffer from depression and/or anxiety and may respond to one kind of health professional and not another. The team in a good pain clinic provides a support mechanism for the patient and also for each other as they pursue their goal of helping the patient at any cost.

Each member of the team who examines a chronic-pain patient meets with the other members to report his findings, and then the team pools its information and insights in order to come to a consensus on the patient's therapy. It is important that the chronic-pain patient receive this type of evaluation because the possibility of an obscure disease or personality disorder being overlooked, or of patient/physician incompatibility interfering with diagnosis and treatment, is greatly reduced.

When a chronic-pain patient visits one specialist, he receives the benefit of that person's skill in his particular field, but his pain may not fall within that realm. There's a much better chance for success in a situation where many specialists are available to cross-check findings. In this setting, the treatment team functions something like a computer, receiving information and processing it to formulate a solution to help the patient achieve his own goal or goals for therapy.

Who comprises the team at a typical multi-disciplinary pain treatment clinic? Let's take a look...

The *neurologist* is a doctor who specializes in diseases of the nervous system. He or she has an intimate knowledge of the role nerves play in the control of muscles and the production of pain. This doctor helps determine if the patient might have a disease, other than a bone problem, that could not be found with X-rays or other anatomical tests.

The *neurosurgeon* is a physician who specializes in *correcting* diseases, injuries and other problems related to the brain and nervous system. Brain surgery is rarely warranted in most types of chronic pain, but if tumors press on nerve centers in the brain, they must be removed. Most of the neurosurgeon's work with chronic-pain patients revolves around his skill and knowledge of the spinal cord and autonomic nervous system.

The *orthopedic surgeon* is a physician who specializes in correcting diseases of the bones, muscles and ligaments. He or she is trained in all aspects of surgery, with specialty training in orthopedic surgery. Highly trained surgeons have had "spine fellowships," during which time they have received extensive training in the surgical correction of spinal or vertebral disorders. Sometimes these surgeons will add metal rods, hooks or plates to stabilize the spine.

The *physiatrist* (physical medicine and rehabilitation medicine—PM & R) is a physician who specializes

133

in the understanding of muscle activity and strength of muscles, tendons and ligaments. He or she is experienced in the area of sports injuries and helping patients recover function after a stroke or surgery.

The *psychologist* is not a physician, so this doctor does not prescribe medication. However, psychologists have specialized training in administering psychological tests and interpreting their results. They also help patients deal with the depression that typically comes with chronic pain, and the feelings of anger that result from chronic and persistent pain. The psychologist also teaches a patient how to relax, either through hypnosis or biofeedback.

The *internist/rheumatologist* is a doctor who understands the biochemistry of the body, and how the body may begin to attack itself, in the form of autoimmune (the body reacting against itself) diseases. Also, prior to any surgery, this type of doctor evaluates a patient to make certain there are no undue risks the surgeon or anesthesiologists should take into consideration.

The *technician* operates the diagnostic equipment found in the pain-clinic setting; for example, he might be a member of the radiology department and therefore be specially trained to handle X-ray equipment. Other technicians specialize in the use of biofeedback machines or thermographic units. The technician is not a physician; nevertheless, he *is* a specialist.

The *psychiatrist* is a physician who specializes in dealing with the emotional problems and mental illness. As a medical doctor, the psychiatrist may prescribe drugs as he or she sees fit. One of the major roles of a psychiatrist (or psychologist) is to *listen* to the problems of the patient and to empathize with them—helping any changes in personality, attitude or behavior they might note, and that might be important to his recovery.

A *physician's assistant* is a licensed practitioner who can provide simple medical services, freeing up the specialists for more complicated medical tasks. On a pain-treatment ward, the physician's assistant might take blood pressures, give injections, palpate sore spots, and report back to the team his impressions of the general health of the patient.

This is just a sampling of the staff members on the pain-clinic team. Different combinations of different specialists and technicians may be available at the various pain clinics around the country. Whatever the combination, all staff members work in concert to help you reach your therapy goals.

Establishing goals is a key undertaking at a pain clinic. If you just visit *a* doctor, his goal will be to stop your complaint of pain by using medication. If you visit *a* surgeon, he will be oriented toward a surgical solution, in order to remove the pain. If you are taking pills, your goal is to relieve the pain. But in the pain clinic, the goal is not necessarily the relief of pain. The goal could be to change attitudes, values or lifestyle, or the goal may be to withdraw you from drugs. This withdrawal may give you more relief in the long run than anything else you may have tried. Whatever the goal, it will not be established by you alone, or by doctors alone, but by a team of which you will be one of the members.

Because each chronic-pain patient suffers in his own way, treatment plans and goals are individualized, tailored to specific needs and perhaps to specific pocketbooks. A treatment course can take anywhere from two weeks to several months to execute and may have to be repeated at another point in time, depending on the severity of the problem. The cost can vary according to whether or not the plan is carried out on an inpatient or outpatient basis. For example, if an operation is called for, treatment plus recuperation and follow-up therapy could take more than several months. Some people need to be readmitted two, three or four times to a pain clinic in order to achieve their goal. Some may be helped on an inpatient basis with a one-week stay. Others may visit the clinic daily for a month while they live at home. All these factors contribute to cost.

A patient may be striving to reach more than one goal. Some patients may set a goal of completing a therapy suggested by the team; some may set an occupational goal for themselves—perhaps learning to tolerate the pain to the point where they can return to work or get a different job to accommodate the limitations imposed on them by their pain.

In some eyes the goal may be minimal, such as setting a recreational directive to attend one of every three family outings. The goal may be a personal one, such as re-establishing a relationship with a family member alienated during the worst of the chronic-pain period in your life.

Once a patient's goals are established, the clinic staff will discuss the situation and use their collective knowledge to formulate a treatment plan to be recommended to the patient. At that point, the patient can choose to participate in the plan or not, as he sees fit. But the staff will explain that failure to take part in the activities suggested can, and probably will, result in the patient not reaching his goals.

Becoming a patient at a pain clinic means making a commitment to your treatment. You cannot just be a receiver of care, prescriptions or operations; you must be an active participant in your treatment plan. You can't reach your goal by sitting on the sidelines.

How do you become a patient at a pain-treatment clinic? The easiest route is through referral by your family physician to a facility in your area. If possible, you then can be seen on an outpatient basis and cut the cost by living at home (only if surgery has been ruled out, of course). If you live too far to commute, it is possible to be hospitalized in a clinic, if bed space is available. Some clinics are associated with teaching hospitals; in these cases, you may be hospitalized in a nearby institution.

Of course, being referred to a pain clinic does not necessarily mean you will become a patient at one. Most clinics are small and bed space is tight. You probably will be interviewed before being taken in.

If you are not placed on a waiting list, the next step before admission to a clinic (in some treatment centers) is a screening examination. Different pain clinics use different screening mechanisms to determine what type of patient they are dealing with. The results from these tests are also used to determine treatment goals and therapy progress. No one is forced to do anything he does not want to do; however, patients who don't fully participate rarely obtain optimal benefits.

While you are undergoing therapy that may include any of the previously listed methods, you also will be taking part in a substantial amount of physical activity designed to improve your overall physical fitness as well as your attitude about the limitations your pain has created. You probably will be walking, climbing stairs, sitting, standing, doing almost anything but stewing about the life of pain you have been leading.

In most clinics, you will not be allowed to talk about your pain except in scheduled therapy sessions. Nurses and other ward personnel are aware of this restriction and will not make conversation with you on the subject of pain. In fact, your verbalization of your pain on the ward will be limited to answering the questions of the physician making rounds or the nurse inquiring about your general health during the day.

You will be asked to do many things despite your complaints of pain. If, for example, you say you cannot walk to the bathroom because of the pain in your legs, the nurse may ask you to take a few steps each day toward the bathroom until you are able to walk there unassisted and without prodding.

Life on the ward will not be luxurious. Your whims will not be catered to, particularly those pertaining to medication. If you are used to swallowing a pill when you feel the pain coming on, you will be forced to do without the painkillers on the ward. You will not be given pain-killers on demand, rather you will receive medication from the staff when they deem it advisable.

You may have visitors, family or friends, but they too will be instructed not to cater to you or to discuss your pain with you, nor will you be allowed to discuss your treatment with them. These restrictions all serve to refocus your thinking. Pain is banished as much as possible from your work, both physically and psychically.

Remember, treating chronic pain is not an emergency. It takes time, just as it took time to erode part of your life. Treatment comes after careful diagnosis, and relief comes only with a change in your attitude. As a patient in a pain-treatment clinic, you must be motivated and certain that you want to get well. Only then will the pain clinic work for you and help you master your suffering.

Ultimately, the time it takes to conquer chronic pain or adjust to it so that you can function as you want to is up to you and to your attitude: no single thing, not the surgeon's knife nor a single magical pill, nor a flow of kind words, will help you manage or eliminate your pain.

In the pain clinic, the treatment begins with belief and trust. The staff proceeds from the belief that the patients who come to them for help are in pain, and it's not just "in their heads." In this way the staff elicits a sense of trust from the patients. Trust is an enormous help when any kind of care is given, but is particularly useful when dealing with chronic-pain patients who often feel as though they've been abandoned along medicine's highway without a friend. With trust, patients are more apt to participate in those recommended treatments that otherwise might have seemed frightening or overwhelming.

Treatments are tailor-made in the pain clinics. No one treatment or combination of therapies is exactly the same for every patient, just as no one's pain is the same as anyone else's.

Treatment ranges from simple withdrawal from drugs to highly complex surgery requiring skill and advanced equipment. All procedures, however, are aimed at treating the *disease* called chronic pain.

## Choosing a Pain Clinic

There are different types of pain clinics, and you should pick one best suited to your needs. So before you select a treatment center, ask yourself the following questions. Your answers will guide you to the proper facility.

1. Has your problem been properly diagnosed? Do you really know what is causing your pain? Do you really *want* to know what is causing your pain? Would you like to know what types of treatments are available to get rid of your pain?

If the answer to any of these questions is "YES," you should consider a "multi-disciplinary diagnostic clinic."

2. Are drugs (narcotics, tranquilizers, alcohol, sleeping pills) a problem? Do you, or does your doctor or someone in your family, think you are addicted to drugs? Have you or someone in your family or friends noticed a change in your personality? Do you notice that you are not as sharp, mentally, as you once were? Do you know what is causing your pain, but just don't know how to deal with it?

If the answer to any of these questions is "YES," then perhaps you should consider an "inpatient behavior-modification clinic."

3. Do you have thoughts of suicide or plans for committing suicide? Are you depressed all the time? Are you argumentative and irritable much of the time? Do you have trouble sleeping or falling asleep most nights but don't know why?

If the answer to any of these questions is "YES," you should consider "inpatient psychiatric hospitalization."

4. Do you not care what is causing your pain, but just want to learn how to cope with it better? Do you want your family to function better, and understand you better? Do you think you are the only one with chronic pain? Do you want to reduce the pain, so that it's a bit more tolerable?

If the answer to any of these questions is "YES," then you should consider an "outpatient pain-treatment center."

Now that you've answered some of the questions about your goals for pain treatment, you can explore the various types of pain clinics available.

MULTI-DISCIPLINARY DIAGNOSTIC CLINIC — This type of clinic has a variety of doctors who work together in an attempt to diagnose what's wrong with you. While there should be just one of these doctors in charge of coordinating your care, you may also be seen by a neurosurgeon, an orthopedic surgeon, an internist, a psychiatrist, a physiatrist or any of the other specialties available depending on the results of their diagnosis and the location of the source of your pain.

Various diagnostic tests may be performed, all of which, in addition to the consultation you may have with other physicians, should be discussed with your coordinating doctor. This doctor should explain to your satisfaction what is wrong with you and what types of treatment are available to you. He should also be able to explain any risks posed by various tests and treatments so you can make an informed decision. When you leave this type of clinic, you should know what to expect from your disease, and what you can do to get help for it. You should also be able to get the type of treatment you need at the very clinic where the diagnosis was made.

INPATIENT BEHAVIORAL-MODIFICATION CLINIC — This type of clinic will usually require you to sign a contract indicating that you will follow the rules of the clinic while a patient there. One essential element of this type of program is the elimination of the use of all harmful medications. Usually, this withdrawal is done in a step-wise fashion so that no discomfort occurs. Also, during treatment, the self-help techniques described in Chapter 6 are utilized and taught to you. Very often, physical therapy is used to increase physical endurance and strength. In some programs, a patient is not permitted to talk about pain, nor permitted to act as if he or she has pain. Usually there is a set program, or a set length of stay, to which the patient must adhere.

INPATIENT PSYCHIATRIC HOSPITALIZATION — A number of researchers have described the psychiatric impact of chronic pain. It is very common, for example, for pain to create depression, sleep disturbance, thoughts of suicide, anger, irritability, anxiety and even suicide attempts. While there are no published figures in this regard, correspondence between researchers at the University of Miami Pain and Rehabilitation Center and the Mensana Clinic indicates that the suicide rate for chronic-pain patients is far higher than that for the general population, perhaps as much as ten times as high. A person should not feel embarrassed or weak if he or she has these feelings, for they are a normal response to chronic pain. The critical thing to understand, however, is the importance of seeking help should feelings of depression or suicide overwhelm you. Depression can be treated and cured. If the depression is severe, accompanied by suicidal plans, it is best treated in a residential hospital setting.

OUTPATIENT PAIN-TREATMENT CENTER — In this type of clinic, the patient uses the self-help techniques described in Chapter 6 to learn how to cope with pain in a manner best suited to his or her own personal needs and goals. There may not be a set program or period of time for treatment, and normally these programs are more flexible than inpatient programs.

*Business Week* magazine, in its January 27, 1992, issue, published a list of the eight best pain clinics in the U.S. They appear here in alphabetical order...

*Cleveland Clinic, Ohio: This is a multi-disciplinary clinic, with emphasis on the evaluation and proper treatment of chronic-pain problems with the goal of improving the quality of the patient's life. Residential and outpatient programs are available.

*Johns Hopkins Hospital Chronic Pain Management Center, Baltimore, Maryland: There are two pain centers at Johns Hopkins Hospital. The outpatient diagnostic service is under the direction of the Department of Neurosurgery, while the inpatient behavioral unit is under the control of psychiatry. The inpatient unit is housed on a locked psychiatric ward. Drug withdrawal and severe depressions are best treated here.

*Mayo Clinic, Rochester, Minnesota: This is a residential program, in a psychiatric setting, which emphasizes improved levels of activity and attitude change toward chronic pain. Drug withdrawal and behavioral modification methods are used to improve the patient's level of functioning.

*Mensana Clinic, Stevenson, Maryland: A multi-disciplinary diagnostic and treatment facility, with inpatient and outpatient services available. In a recent study here, fifty percent of the facility's patients were found to have surgically correctable problems.

*New York Pain Treatment Program, New York: The belief at this clinic is that chronic pain itself, regardless of the cause, is a disease. Hypnosis and other self-help techniques are employed to help a patient cope with the pain and improve his or her life.

*Pain Control and Rehabilitation Institute of Georgia, Atlanta: This unit is primarily a behavior modification center with an emphasis on physical therapy and self-help training.

*University of Miami Pain and Rehabilitation Center, Florida: This is a residential behavior-modification program emphasizing vigorous and strenuous physical therapy with all efforts directed at improving a patient's level of activity.

*University of Washington Pain Treatment Center, Seattle: The nation's oldest pain clinic was established in 1953 by J.J. Bonica, M.D., the founder and past president of the International Society for the Study of Pain. This is a strong behavioral-modification program with an emphasis on improving levels of activity and the quality of life. It is primarily a residential unit, although some outpatient treatment is available.

## A Pain Victim's Odyssey

It may be helpful for you to see what it's like to be a victim of chronic pain—to seek help and to fail to find it. Sometimes the trail can end in disaster and financial ruin, or sometimes it can lead to the therapy that brings relief. The woman in the following account was fortunate; her quest ended at a pain clinic.

Harriet is twenty-four years old. She worked very hard for two years after high school to save enough money to put toward the entrance fee and tuition payments in a nursing program. Harriet's lifelong dream was to become a registered nurse, wear the profession's white uniform and help sick people. Even as a child, when Harriet play-acted, she was a nurse.

Harriet was like a whirlwind in her nursing program, running from class to class, working after school to keep up with the tuition payments and trying to enjoy some sort of social life by accepting an occasional casual date on weekends. Harriet's only regret was that she had to live at home instead of in the dormitory with the other nursing students: the money she saved on room and board went to incidental school expenses.

Harriet's whirlwind came to a painful stop the day after she wore a brand new pair of crepe-sole nursing shoes she bought on sale. The shoes didn't fit exactly right, but she liked how they looked. Harriet wore them all day on the ward, and they pinched and rubbed her feet until she developed several painful blisters. Even though she did not wear the shoes the next day and her blisters were all bandaged, her left foot continued to throb.

Harriet thought she might have pulled a muscle from foolishly walking in tight shoes, and she tried to ignore the pain. But after a week the throbbing still hadn't disappeared, forcing Harriet to curtail her part-time job and ward work .

Several weeks later her foot was so painful that she couldn't wear stockings and was unable to put any weight on the toes of her left foot. She hobbled to her classes as carefully as she could, but doing so was at best a waste of time for she couldn't listen to lectures, she couldn't concentrate, and she didn't feel like taking notes. At worst, going to class was extremely trying and painful.

Harriet became even more determined to ignore the pain and asked a fellow student to accompany her to the student health clinic so should could get a pair of crutches, hoping they would enable her to keep her weight off the painful foot and perhaps make it easier for her to get to classes without feeling exhausted. The friend said she'd help Harriet get the crutches, but insisted she see a doctor in the student health service.

Harriet told the attending physician about the problem with her foot. At first the physician suspected that Harriet's pain was caused by thrombophlebitis, an inflammation of the major veins in the legs and the same ailment that attacked President Richard Nixon during his final days in office, when he had to take frequent rests and keep his foot up on a stool. The doctor ordered a phlebogram for Harriet. She spent several days in the hospital waiting for the results. They finally came back negative.

Harriet told her doctor that lately she'd been very depressed, and that she was feeling anxious about the possibility of missing final exams—so anxious, in fact, that she'd been having dreams about it. She told the doctor she was desperate to get rid of the pain, not only because it hurt but even more because it prevented her from doing the things she wanted and felt needed to be done.

Although the doctor prescribed several potent narcotic painkillers and sleeping pills, Harriet's pain did not clear up and continued to interfere with her activity by making her immobile. After several weeks of observation in the student clinic, her condition had become so bad that water splashing on her thigh from a sponge bath was enough to cause her considerable pain.

The student health physician called in an orthopedic surgeon, who immediately gave Harriet a complete series of examinations. The surgeon could find nothing wrong in any of these tests and so suggested that a psychiatric evaluation might be in order. She felt that Harriet might be overreacting to the pressures of school combined with the emotional stress of working on a ward for the first time.

The psychiatrist referred Harriet to a pain clinic near the school campus where she had an office.

On her admission, the staff of the pain-treatment center asked Harriet a series of questions to determine how she felt in general and how she thought the pain altered her lifestyle.

They found Harriet to be a highly motivated young lady who had goals set for herself and was depressed because achieving them seemed to be so far in the future, when only a few months before they had seemed so close at hand. They also discovered that Harriet was angry with doctors—she felt they didn't believe she was in pain. She did not trust them anymore because she felt that they didn't trust her to be honest with them. She was also upset because she got the distinct feeling that the student health physician thought she was faking her pain to get attention or to get out of taking her final exams.

Harriet was indulging in some self-pity, the staff decided, feeling sorry for herself because she believed she might never realize her dream of being a nurse, but most of all, Harriet was miserable. She was distressed by the pain and because all the pills prescribed for her made her feel groggy and robbed her of her ability to think sharply, a talent she considered to be one of her most precious possessions.

Harriet received a complete physical exam and filled out a medical history for the pain center records.

The internist in charge of her physical looked at her legs several times and found that her left foot was mildly swollen (edema), mostly about the toes. Her left leg also seemed to be cooler to the touch than her lower right leg. When he tried to examine her left leg more closely, Harriet told him he was causing her a great deal of sharp, shooting pain. The internist then asked Harriet to stand up and place weight on both her legs equally. Harriet did this with difficulty. She could not fully extend her left knee. Otherwise, Harriet appeared to be a healthy young woman.

Because of the marked difference in temperature between her lower left leg and right one, the internist ordered a thermographic exam, in which, as explained in Chapter 5, areas of pain can be mapped out by their decreased temperature compared to normal tissue temperature. The thermograph showed a generalized coldness from her foot to her calf in her left leg as compared to the right leg. The lower left leg was as much as two degrees centigrade cooler (an average temperature difference in positive findings in thermography). The thermographic map of the painful area suggested there was some damage to a sympathetic nerve in her leg.

Harriet checked into the pain clinic as an inpatient. She agreed to follow the rules of the clinic and signed a "contract" with the staff regarding her participation. The physician in charge informed he about the possible sympathetic nerve damage, explaining in lay terms what it meant. He suggested that she try a lumbar sympathetic block (a block to nerves in the lower regions of the back). Harriet agreed.

The blocks were performed at the pain clinic by an anesthesiologist. Harriet had immediate relief from her pain.

When the effect of the block wore off and the pain returned, Harriet returned to the clinic. The pain clinic once again recommended a lumbar sympathetic block, which again was successful.

Following this procedure, the staff psychiatrist, anesthesiologist, internist and social worker got together and discussed Harriet's case. They felt she would be a good candidate for a sympathectomy, a surgical severing of the nerve that was causing her pain (as indicated by the success of blocking that nerve). Harriet had proved to be a motivated patient with a good premorbid adjustment who showed signs of trying to cope with and adjust to the pain, but was frustrated in her efforts.

After explaining the benefits and risks of the surgery to Harriet, the staff recommended that she have the operation. Harriet agreed. She had immediate relief from the pain and went on to finish her studies.

She returned to the pain clinic two years later for a follow-up study of her progress. The new thermograph showed that her lower left leg was a full 2.5 degrees warmer than it had been during her period of pain.

Harriet went on to receive her degree and achieve her dream of working as a registered nurse—a busy one who walks all day without discomfort. She also wears shoes that fit.

Not all patients who enter the pain clinic are as successful as Harriet. It is true that some people never receive complete relief from pain. The staff continues to support them, however, and to help them in every way they can to be active and function to their fullest.

# 8

*O*ne of the primary goals of a pain-treatment center is to change the patient's behavior with respect to his pain. Because the pain over time has slowly altered the patient's behavior and then affected everything he does, the clinic staff must try to change that behavior so the pain is no longer the focus of the patient's life.

Behavior is the manner in which a person responds to his environment—when he is alone or among other people. Behavior modification is a system of altering behavior by a variety of means.

Operant (Skinnerian) conditioning is a form of behavior modification that is used in some clinics: if the behavior exhibited is considered desirable, a reward is given; when behavior that is undesirable is displayed, a punishment is given to discourage a repeat performance. In other words, an outside force, whoever is dispensing the rewards or punishments, is changing the behavior, rather than the patient changing his behavior solely on his own.

The classic experiment in this type of conditioning involved Pavlov's dog, who was taught to salivate at the sound of a bell. Whenever the caged animal heard a bell, he was immediately given a piece of food. This action was repeated often enough so that the dog salivated whenever he heard a bell, wherever he was.

In the pain clinic, before a system of rewards and punishments can be set up, the staff must determine what each individual's desirable and undesirable behavior is. In general, desirable behavior leads to the goals that patient and staff members mutually establish at the patient's admission, and undesirable behavior contributes to the patient's fixation on pain.

For example, undesirable behavior for pain-clinic patients is talking about the pain at any time except when asked a specific question by the physician or other medical personnel. So if you start a conversation with a ward nurse about your pain, "My leg is really bothering me today; I don't think I'll get up and make my bed, and I also would like some more of that medication Dr. R. prescribed last week," the nurse will mete out "punishment"—she will ignore the statement.

Generally, if someone says something and is ignored, he will not repeat the statement. Being ignored causes embarrassment and frustration, both of which are unpleasant feelings that most people like to avoid. As a result, when the nurse and others continually ignore statements about your pain, you will avoid making them, and instead make statements that will lead to a conversational response. The punishment meted out reduces those forms of behavior the staff wants you to avoid—your behavior has been modified.

On the other hand, if you exhibit a behavior on the ward that brings you closer to your goal, such as stretching your arm during a physical therapy session (when you have kept that arm immobile for many months), you will be verbally encouraged to continue that behavior. Encouragement is also accompanied by praise. For example, if you willingly follow the therapist's instructions and go a bit further than asked, she will praise you. Most people like praise—it acts as a reward. You will continue to try to win the praise (the reward) by doing just a little bit more for the therapist. By reinforcing what she has observed to be a good behavior in you, the therapist has helped you to modify your behavior. You no longer keep your arm immobile and you have moved a little further on the path to your goal.

Most activities on the ward are fashioned to encourage modification of the chronic-pain patient's behavior. Making your bed, going to the nurses' station for your medication or simply socializing by chatting with fellow patients are all behaviors that are encouraged. They are activities that will keep you functioning and lead you to a life outside your pain.

Behavior modification actually is the beginning of a new way of life. Its purpose is to remove pain from your life as much as possible. If your behavior changes are successful, you reap all the rewards. You achieve other goals. Refocusing your thoughts and activities need not be the only end of behavior modification. You will relate to people differently if the method is successful. Relating to people differently, you will feel less depressed, better about yourself, and you will probably start believing that you can learn to tolerate your pain.

Motivation to achieve these goals is most clearly seen in this phase of treatment. The patient must have a sincere desire to be pain free or a sincere desire to resume a normal life in order for behavior modification to truly work. The patient who is so motivated has a good chance for successful treatment.

The pain clinic, in some ways, can be compared to the therapeutic community concept. The therapeutic community is an alternative to placing drug abusers or alcoholics in jails or prisons. The whole purpose of the community, which is composed of a group of people with a common need and goal (to get off drugs and remain drug free), is therapy. Every activity in the community is therapy. The therapy teaches the residents responsibility. They need to learn to be responsible for their own lives, as they forfeited that responsibility when they became addicted to drugs. Drug addiction is in part a lifestyle, so the therapeutic community shows the addict that there can be a different lifestyle that is fulfilling and useful.

With its behavior-modification program, the pain clinic also strives to teach the chronic-pain patient to take responsibility for his life and his health, rather than focusing on his disease. This should enable the patient to discard his former perceptions about the pain—of course, this all occurs in tandem with the other treatments the pain clinic offers.

Not that you have to go to a pain clinic to practice behavior modification. For example, if you find yourself avoiding a party because the pain puts a damper on your spirits, make a special effort to go in spite of how you feel. You may have a good time and manage to forget the pain.

If you find you are doing less and less of what you want to do, get yourself a small notebook and write down what you have avoided doing when you feel the pain. Do this for several weeks. Then look back at your notes, pick an activity that seems easy and work at doing it the next time you feel the pain. Pick one activity at a time until you have tried them all again. You may have started coping with your chronic pain.

# 9

## RELIEF WITHOUT ADDICTION

*T*his chapter is about drug management: why certain drugs are selected to alleviate pain, how they work and how physicians determine which ones to use for each patient. To aid in your understanding of this subject, we begin with the following list of the basic categories of drugs and their effects on your body. The categories are not rigid and in some cases a drug will fit into several of them.

### Analgesics

Analgesics are drugs that relieve or allay pain. They range from simple and ubiquitous aspirin to potent narcotics defined as substances that produce euphoria in addition to pain relief. Narcotics are habituating and can be addictive with long-term use.

### Minor Tranquilizers

These tranquilizers are drugs that have a calming effect; they produce a peaceful feeling without inducing sleep. However, they can cause depression and rage reactions and alter sleep patterns. And they are usually addicting.

### Major Tranquilizers

There are five major classes of drugs in this category. They are used to control psychotic behavior but can also be good antianxiety agents when taken in small doses. They are not addicting, but some can create shaking hands or lip tremor, usually controllable or reversible if detected early enough.

### Hypnotics and Sedatives

These drugs produce a calming effect while they induce sleep. They usually are addicting and alter natural sleep. Barbiturates are among the most common sedatives, and they also act as hypnotics and are addicting.

### Stimulants

Stimulants are drugs that increase or speed up the functions and activities of the central nervous system. The amphetamines are the most common stimulants, and they also act as appetite suppressants for about two weeks. They are habituating and can cause depression with long use. Caffeine is a widely used stimulant.

### Antidepressants or Mood Elevators

These are relatively new drugs with the power to alter mood. Such drugs are prescribed to combat anxiety and fight off depression. They are not addicting or habituating, but some have uncomfortable side effects.

### Hallucinogens
These drugs primarily produce hallucinations and as yet have not been found to have a medical purpose.

### Muscle Relaxants
These are a specific group of drugs that reduce muscle spasms created by certain pain states. Some minor and major tranquilizers can also act as muscle relaxants.

### Anti-inflammatory Agents
Beginning with aspirin and incorporating a host of steroids and steroid-like drugs, these agents reduce the swelling that can be associated with some chronic pain. The major side effect is stomach upset.

### Vasoactive Compounds
These substances are designed to permit increased blood flow to damaged areas by enlarging the diameter of blood vessels. Some of these drugs are useful for the treatment of headache.

### Anti-Convulsants
These drugs are designed to quiet the action of the nerves and can also be used to reduce nerve pain. Some have potentially fatal side effects.

In an effort to kill their pain, many patients spend years experimenting with a variety of therapies and physicians, and nothing works. During their long and fruitless search for a solution, many become addicted to drugs.

Addiction is a physical dependence on drugs; your body craves them and requires that you take them. The body becomes accustomed to drugs and needs them as it needs air and water. Because addiction causes chemical changes, the body will experience withdrawal symptoms without the substances on which it has come to depend. These symptoms can include shakes, sweats, cramps and convulsions. Long-term use of addictive drugs can lead to altered personality, depression and, in some cases, permanent residual brain damage.

Because of these undesirable side effects, narcotics and the minor tranquilizers such as Valium and Librium, all of which have addictive potential, should not be considered the most beneficial analgesics on the market shelves. Yet they are the most frequently prescribed for chronic pain. What other drugs, then, can or should be used to reduce pain, anxiety and depression? The answer to this question is directly related to what you have learned in previous chapters about the many factors that cause pain and affect one's perception of it.

## Anxiety and Pain

One of the variables that must be taken into account when a physician prescribes a drug for acute pain is to what extent the patient's anxiety may be intensifying his pain. More than forty years ago, one of the earliest pain researchers, Edward K. Beecher, M.D., studied acute pain and how it affected individuals in different locations and settings. He chose as his subjects a group of men who had been in combat and lay wounded on a battlefield. Because their injuries were so extensive, these soldiers had to be evacuated from the combat zone. The wounds varied in severity and involved different parts of the body, including chest and stomach wounds as well as multiple-fractured bones.

Dr. Beecher matched the soldiers' wounds to similar injuries sustained by a group of civilians who then needed to undergo major surgery in a hospital. The civilians also had chest and stomach wounds and compounded fractures.

Dr. Beecher found that the soldiers were less likely to request morphine than their civilian counterparts. He decided that the perception of acute pain, how much pain was felt or how much pain the patients were aware of, depended largely on how they perceived their immediate environment.

To the civilians, surgery meant disaster, being removed from comfortable and familiar objects at home and placed in a frightening and sterile hospital. It meant coming face to face with the fact that they were ill, and this made the patients anxious.

For the soldiers, having surgery meant getting off the life-threatening battlefield to the relative comforts and safety of a hospital. It meant getting help for their wounds, and most of all, it meant getting out of war. The prospect of being evacuated to a field hospital for surgery was welcome. Therefore the soldiers did not experience the anxiety of their civilian counterparts, and according to Dr. Beecher, because of the reduced anxiety they perceived less pain. The evidence for this was that the soldiers made fewer requests for narcotics before surgery.

Dr. Beecher's theories about the effect of anxiety on the perception of pain were borne out by other researchers who found that a quantity of Thorazine, a potent tranquilizer used to calm violent mental patients, is equally effective in reducing postoperative pain as a slightly smaller dose of morphine. Thorazine does not have any of the analgesic power of morphine. Why then did the Thorazine work? It worked because of its calming effect.

According to many physicians, a great deal of postoperative pain is due to the patient's anxiety and general nervousness about the outcome of surgery. When patients enter surgery, they are anxious about the entire procedure. Some of the best surgeons are those who establish rapport with their patients, who talk to the patients prior to surgery—explaining at length what is going to happen to them, what techniques are going to be used, and what the patient should expect of himself after the surgery. Because knowing what to expect offers some measure of security, these patients are relatively calm going into the operating room and come out requesting less painkiller.

Looking at the result these investigators achieved, it would seem that the physician should be able to avoid the use of narcotic analgesics—which are harmful when administered for long periods of time—if he can reduce his patient's anxiety, whether treating acute or chronic pain.

What drugs should be substituted for narcotics? Ideally, the chemical should fight anxiety, which eliminates some of the emotional components of pain, and have some pain reducing powers all of its own, without being addicting.

The phenothiazines are one such category of drug. Though they too have side effects, they are not nearly as severe in consequence as those of the benzodiazepines. For example, a physician might prescribe Valium as a tranquilizer hoping to reduce his patient's stress and anxiety about pain by calming him. However, the patient may become depressed, or may in fact have a paradoxical increase in his pain, due to the Valium (because of its chemical action) and the physician may eventually recommend that he see a psychiatrist because of these reactions. The psychiatrist may take the patient off Valium, and the patient may report either a lifting of depression, or a lessening of the pain. This phenomenon can be attributed to the action of Valium upon a drug in the brain called serotonin. Valium blocks the release of serotonin, which interferes with natural sleep, reduces the body's ability to tolerate pain, and, in some cases, may cause depression.

The phenothiazine tranquilizers are more effective against chronic pain, and have fewer potentials for depressive side effects. They are effective because they block receptor sites for two other chemicals in the brain (dopamine and norepinephrine) and the blocking of norepinephrine (nor-adrenalin) receptor sites increases pain tolerance. In doing this they also combat anxiety when administered in small doses. However, they too have side effects, such as restlessness and abnormal movements, and should be used with caution on a long-term basis.

## Depression and Drugs

The use of antidepressant medication for chronic pain is a relatively new but promising application of these drugs. There are basically three types of antidepressant medications available. These are the tricyclic antidepressants, monoamine oxidase inhibitors, and psychostimulants.

Depression is thought to be caused in some people by a chemical imbalance, specifically a deficiency of the neurotransmitters norepinephrine and serotonin. Therefore, it would appear that if these substances could be increased in the central nervous system, the depression could be alleviated.

It is now possible to biochemically differentiate two types of depression: first, a depression caused by a reduction of a drug in the brain called serotonin, and second, a depression caused by the reduction of the drug norepinephrine which, as noted above, is also in the brain. A reduction of either of these drugs may be accomplished by several means. Their receptor site activity can be artificially blocked by the administration of certain drugs, such as those used to treat high blood pressure. Or, the stores of these chemicals in the brain can be depleted by the use of other drugs, notably reserpine-containing compounds, which again are applied to the treatment of high blood pressure. Certain chemicals, such as Valium, can inhibit the release of serotonin, thereby causing depression, altered sleep patterns, and increased sensation of pain.

The *tricyclic antidepressants* reduce depression by increasing certain neurosynaptic transmitters (the chemicals in the brain of which we have recently talked—

serotonin, norepinephrine and dopamine). However, not all tricyclic antidepressants have the same effect, because they work on different neurosynaptic transmitters.

As discussed in Chapter 2, sensory nerves, such as pain fibers, are stimulated by the experience of a pain-producing sensation or event, such as extremes of temperature, pressure and irritation. This stimulation is transmitted by a series of electrical impulses that travel along the nerve and cause the release of a chemical from the nerve ending. This chemical, which is called a neurosynaptic transmitter, or neurotransmitter (such as serotonin, norepinephrine or dopamine), then takes over. The neurosynaptic transmitter jumps across a gap between two nerves (a synapse), binds to a specific receptor site on an adjacent nerve, and then chemically stimulates it to begin a series of electrical impulses along this second nerve. In less than a thousandth of a second this chemical is reabsorbed by the nerve that released it, and its action is thereby ended.

The important concept here is the specificity of these chemicals for one nerve or the other. As you can imagine, merely applying electrical current excites all types of nerves. However, by applying certain specific chemicals, one can excite or chemically block one type of nerve or another.

A moderate portion of this reabsorbed chemical is digested or used (metabolized) by the cell; it is broken down with the help of another chemical, or enzyme. This chemical is called monoamine oxidase.

All this brings us to *monoamine-oxidase inhibitors*. These chemicals work as antidepressants by increasing the concentration of available neurotransmitters—by inhibiting their metabolism by monoamine oxidase. If neurotransmitters are not metabolized, there will be more of them. If there are more of them, depression resulting from a deficiency of neurotransmitters can be relieved. Since the neurotransmitters serotonin and norepinephrine both are metabolized by monoamine oxidase, the monoamine-oxidase inhibitors allow the buildup of both chemical transmitters.

*Psychostimulants* function differently from the tricyclic and monoamine-oxidase-inhibitor-type antidepressants. They work by increasing the concentration of the desired neurotransmitter in the synapse by stimulating the release of the neurosynaptic transmitter from the pre-synaptic cell. In stimulating the release of the neurotransmitter, they generally stimulate the central nervous system. This is due to the release of a chemical called norepinephrine. This chemical in high concentration in the brain has been shown to increase the perception of pain. After a while, they can deplete the brain's supply of norepinephrine, and cause depression, or even a psychotic episode that looks like paranoid schizophrenia. Psychostimulants, therefore, are not the drug of first or even second choice to combat depression.

Rather than stimulate the chronic-pain patient's system, the physician wishes to sedate it to some degree, and the phenothiazine tranquilizers work well for this purpose. Within this group of tranquilizers are a subdivision that are especially effective for chronic-pain patients and have fewer sedative side effects than other drugs within this category. Drugs such as Stelazine, Prolixin and Trilafon have less chance of producing drowsy, groggy side effects. Another drug that is not a phenothiazine, but in a completely different drug category, Haldol, has even fewer sedative side effects. However, the basic mechanism of action is the same. These drugs all work by blocking the post-synaptic reception of dopamine and norepinephrine. It has recently been shown that the blocking of norepinephrine lessens the perception of pain, and therefore produces some degree of relief.

Combinations of certain tricyclic antidepressants and some phenothiazines that do not have a sedative effect have been found useful for the treatment of pain from post-herpetic neuralgia and intractable cancer. Research by Dr. Arthur Taub at Yale University has been confirmed by a variety of other investigators, which has led to the widespread use of the combination of Elavil and Prolixin.

Aspirin, of course, is one of the most common painkillers in the world, and it is most effective for the treatment of pain from arthritis. Scientists as yet do not know exactly how it kills pain, but they suspect that it somehow activates the release of a substance called prostaglandin H, which acts as an analgesic at the pain nerve-fiber (free nerve endings). Unfortunately, too much aspirin can cause another type of pain—gastritis (stomach pain). This can be avoided by using a buffered compound that does not irritate the stomach lining as much as aspirin. (Scientists make breakthroughs in the arthritis field all the time and recently have announced some success with the use of lasers—powerful concentrations of pencil-thin light—in the fight against the pain of rheumatoid arthritis.)

Some chemicals when inhaled can cause facial pain. This pain can be combated by anti-inflammatory drugs.

It is very difficult to relieve the pain of a patient who is dying from cancer or another disease that causes him to live in pain that can last for several years. Not too long ago, doctors were afraid to addict the dying patient who suffered a great deal of agonizing pain. They felt that to give them too much morphine, Demerol, Talwin or Codeine would be wrong, because it could only lead to narcotic addiction. In recent years, however, attitudes about the dying have changed, and so has the attitude toward a more liberal use of narcotics for these patients.

In an attempt to avoid addiction some physicians experimented with the "P.R.N." concept. P.R.N. are the initials for the words per required need (administer as needed). In other words, the patient suffering from terminal bone cancer could not receive his medication until his last dose of narcotics had worn off and he was in pain again and needed the drugs.

Much of the cancer patient's pain was probably due to the anxiety of anticipation: waiting to be hit with the pain again, hoping it wouldn't happen, tensing up because he knew it would. When physicians follow a fixed timetable for the administration of the drug, giving it to the patient every four hours, or preferably every three hours, since the effect of most narcotics lasts only two to three hours, the patient no longer anxiously awaits for the pain to hit again—because it won't. It will be stopped before the last dose of medication wears off. With his anxiety reduced, the patient's perception of pain also is reduced. In fact, doctors prescribing drugs on the fixed timetable find that their patients actually need fewer narcotics to maintain them in a pain-free state, rather than more, the "more" that leads to addiction.

American practitioners also have begun following in the footsteps of their counterparts in Britain, who for many years have given their terminal patients living in pain a "cocktail" whose ingredients include a narcotic, a stimulant, alcohol and flavoring. This combination of drugs allows the patient to be pain free (the narcotic) while remaining alert (the stimulant), and the medication is made palatable by its flavoring.

Among the most promising drugs on the horizon are the body's own opiates, the endorphines and enkephalines (mentioned in Chapter 2). If the physician can learn to stimulate the natural opiates into action, he will be able to alleviate pain without the use of harmful drugs. The key to stimulating these drugs, however, is not known, but there are suggestions that the use of electrical stimulation, or acupuncture-like techniques may excite their production.

The following is a list of the most commonly prescribed drugs for chronic pain and an explanation of their basic action. (The list of brand names does not imply endorsement.)

### Analgesics

Aspirin, buffered aspirin and aspirin compounds are all over-the-counter drugs that are effective in combating headaches, muscular aches and pains, arthritis, sinusitis, and the aches and pains due to fatigue from overexertion. The buffered compounds contain an antacid to protect the stomach lining from the effects of aspirin. Many of the products contain caffeine, which acts as a diuretic and a general brain stimulant.

### Aspirin Products
Alka-Seltzer Effervescent Pain Reliever®
Alka-Seltzer Plus Cold Medicine®
Arthritis Strength Bufferin®
Ascriptin®
Bayer Aspirin®
Bayer Children's Aspirin®
Bayer Children's Cold Tablets®
Bufferin®
Congesprin®
Cope®
Coricidin®
Empirin Compound®
Excedrin®
Excedrin P.M.®
Vanquish®

### Narcotics
Narcotics, some of which are derivatives of opium, are the most potent painkillers, and they are addictive.

The following narcotics are administered alone with aspirin or aspirin-type compounds for the relief of all pain in all degrees of severity. If they prove ineffective, the only stronger drug is morphine.
Ascriptin with Codeine®
Demerol Hydrochloride®
Dilaudid Hydrochloride®
Empirin Compound with Codeine Phosphate®

Emprazil-C Tablets®
Pavadon Elixir®
Percodan®
Sublimaze®
Tylenol with Codeine Tablets®

These narcotics are synthetics in combination with other chemicals.

Darvon®
Levoprome®
Talwin Compound®

The following are local anesthetics, used to produce a temporary state of numbing. These are the kinds of substances used in blocks.

Marcaine®
Novocaine®
Xylocaine Hydrochloride®

## Anti-inflammatory Agents

These drugs help fight pain by reducing swelling. The swelling may be caused by a variety of diseases, including gout, arthritis and muscle damage.

Ansaid®
Benemid®
Colchicine®
Feldene®
Indocin®
Motrin®
Napersin®
Naprosyn®
Orudis®

Telectin®
Tolectin®
Toridol®
Volterin®
Zyloprim®

## Anti-Convulsant Drugs

These drugs fight pain by quieting the action of the nerves. There are several different mechanisms by which a drug may exert anti-convulsant activity, but for the sake of simplicity, the drugs of this category are listed by their end result, not how they accomplish this end.

Depakene (Depakote)®
Diamox®
Dilantin®
Klonopin®
Mysolin®
Tegretol®

## Antidepressants (or Mood Elevators)

These drugs work by reducing depression, and in some cases relieving anxiety. As mentioned in the chapter, they also work directly on the mechanisms of chronic pain.

Drugs working primarily on serotonin augmentation:

Adapin®
Anafranil®
Desyrel®
Elavil®
Prozac®
Sinequan®

Wellbutrin®
Zoloft®
Drugs that work both on serotonin and norepi-
nephrine:
    Imipramine Hydrochloride Tablets®
    Tofranil Ampuls®
    SK-Pramine Tablets®
    Drugs that work primarily on norepinephrine:
    Aventyl®
    Desipramine®
    Norpramine®
    Vivactil®

### Hypnotics and Sedatives

In low dosages, these drugs provide a calming effect, usually associated with drowsy side effects, while at higher dosages, these drugs induce a non-natural sleep. Most of the drugs listed below are addictive, interfere with the normal pattern of sleep, suppress the ability to dream, and may cause withdrawal symptoms upon the cessation of their use.

    Aquachloral Supprettes®
    Dalmane®
    Luminal®
    Placidyl®

#### BARBITURATES

    Alurate®
    Amytal®
    Butisol Sodium Elixir, Tablets®
    Dialog®
    Eskabarb Spansule Capsules®

Luminal®
Mebaral®
Nembutal Elixir®
Repan®
Seconal Elixir®
Tuinal®

**NON-BARBITURATES**
Dalmane®
Halcion®
Placidyl®
Prosom®
Restoril®
Tranxene®

## Minor Tranquilizers, or Benzodiazepines

These drugs have a sedative and hypnotic effect. Some of these drugs also act to alter moods, may be addicting, and can cause depression. They have little or no use in the treatment of chronic pain.

Ativan®
Azine®
Halcion®
Librax®
Librium Capsules®
Serax®
Tranxene®
Valium®
Xanax®

## Major Tranquilizers, or Phenothiazines and their Combinations

These drugs are not without their side effects, but they do inhibit the neurosynaptic transmitters, and can be useful in combating anxiety. They include Phenothiazines, Buterophenones, Phioxanthines, Molindones and Dibenzoxazepines.

PHENOTHIAZINES

Compazine®
Mellaril®
Prolixin®
Serentil®
Stelazine®
Thorazine®
Trilafon®
Vesprin®

Major Tranquilizers with Phenothiazine-Like Action
(BUTEROPHENONES, PHIOXANTHINES, MOLINDONES, DIBENZOXAZEPINES)

Haldol®
Loxitane®
Moban®
Navane®

## Stimulants

These drugs increase the action of the central nervous system. They often are prescribed to counter the effects of sedative actions of analgesics.

**AMPHETAMINES**
Benzedrine Sulfate®
Biphetamine®
Desoxyn®
Dexamyl®
Dexedrine®
Didrex®
Eskatrol®

**NONAMPHETAMINES**
Sanorex®
Tenuate®
Tepanil®

## Muscle Relaxants

These drugs reduce muscle spasms created by certain pain states.
Flexeril®
Lioresil®
Parafon Forte®
Robaxin®
Skelaxin®
Soma®
Valium Tablets® (a benzodiazepine, which may worsen pain)

## Vasoactive Compounds

These drugs permit more blood to flow to damaged areas by increasing the diameter of blood vessels. They can be useful in treating headache pain.
Calan®
Cardizem®

Corgard®
Cyclospasmol®
Gynergin®
Inderal®
Nicobid®
Octin®
Regitine®
Rogaine®
Tenormin®
Verapamil®
Verlan®

# 10

## PAIN AND THE FAMILY

*A*s chronic pain takes center stage in the life of its victims, so too the chronic-pain patient becomes the focus of his family; he demands attention. His complaints disturb everyone in the household. His schedule of pills or doctor's examinations burdens the schedules of others and probably breaks the family's budget. Resentment builds. If family members do not cater to him, or if they try to ignore his constant indisposition and protestations of imminent collapse, the patient resents the "unfair" way he feels he is being treated. The family members, in turn, resent the amount of time the patient demands; they can understand that he doesn't feel well, but eventually they come to believe that he could feel better and contribute more to the household if he truly wanted to. Chronic pain has the potential to destroy its victim's family as well as its victim.

Karen is a bright young woman who has always thought of herself as independent. As soon as she finished high school she said good-bye to her family and set off on a cross-country tour of Europe on her own, hitchhiking all the way, against family advice. When she returned to this country, she decided to see it the same way and took another year before she settled down in a small apartment in her hometown. She decided to go to junior college, and her father offered to pay her tuition.

As soon as she finished school, she went into business for herself designing and producing greeting cards. She enjoyed what she was doing so much that she decided to do everything for herself, so she also started selling the cards, replacing her brother who had helped her with this part of the business. Both aspects of the work appealed to her—the artistic end appealed to her creative nature; selling her cards gave her an outlet for her aggressiveness.

Though Karen considered herself a loner, she accepted a marriage proposal from a department-store executive who had proposed not too long after she had sold him a batch of her greeting cards. Joe was an old-fashioned sort who insisted that his wife not work and that she settle down and raise all the children they planned to have. Karen fought him on this until the day their first child was born, and then they reached a compromise. Karen would move her business into the house and simultaneously be a businesswoman and a full-time mother, as Joe felt she should be.

After two more children in as many years, Karen couldn't find much time for her business, and it started to fail. Just about the time Karen's business started doing poorly, she began to wake up in the morning with low-back pain. Karen and Joe decided that their semisoft mattress was the culprit and decided to buy a firmer one, but the harder mattress didn't help.

For the next few years, while she traveled from doctor to doctor looking for relief, Karen was also trying to salvage her business. Eventually she was spending little time at home and moved her business back to an office building in the city. The move was accomplished only after some vicious arguments between her and Joe and a promise from Karen that all her free time would be spent with the children.

In addition to her emotional clashes with Joe over her business, the back pain kept on giving her trouble. It began to interfere with her sex life to the point where she told Joe that it was better for her if they had no sex at all, because the pain was too much to bear. Karen always seemed pressed for time. She felt tremendously guilty about neglecting her children while trying to re-establish her business—and felt angry about feeling guilty. She was also fatigued from the pain, which prevented her from getting a good night's sleep. Karen's pain was fighting Joe and the three children for her attention—and winning.

But what about Joe and the three children: Where did they fit into Karen's life, particularly Karen's life marred by chronic pain?

By the time a psychiatrist referred Karen to a pain-treatment center, Joe was ready to leave her. He had often thought about disappearing one day and making a new life for himself in another state under a different name.

Joe was fed up with Karen and her pain. All he ever heard when he was home was that Karen didn't feel well and wanted to be left alone. He argued with her all the time. He felt that she was a rotten mother and a worse wife. He felt that during the past few years (since she had rekindled her business) she had become enormously self-centered and was ignoring everybody.

During the heat of one of their arguments, he finally told her that he didn't believe she was really in pain. He told her that he felt it was just an excuse to stay away from him. Karen admitted she thought he had been running around with other women—he had before when she was pregnant—so she didn't see what difference it made to him that they were no longer having sex. Joe exploded when she said that and nearly hit her, but instead he left the house for two weeks. He told himself he just didn't want to hear about her pain anymore.

When he returned home, Karen suggested that they both enter family therapy at the pain-treatment center. Joe agreed. After their first meeting, the therapist requested that Karen and Joe bring the children to the sessions. He felt that Karen's pain probably had affected them, and that their behavior, in turn, probably had an effect on Karen, and on her pain.

During therapy Joe admitted that he felt left out of Karen's life, ignored and abused. He said that he understood that Karen's back hurt her, but on another level and after two years, he just couldn't believe that she really was in pain anymore. Believing this made him angry and made him want "to get even" with Karen for deceiving him, by hurting her and making her angry. Joe said he felt as if he were being pulled apart by his emotions, and he thought that the best thing for him to do would be to leave Karen permanently. He said that he saw no alternative to leaving, that most of his sympathy for Karen had been eroded by their quarrels and her complaints about pain.

The children appeared to be as upset as Joe over their mother's pain and her behavior. The children were young (ages eight, nine, and ten), but articulate. They all said that they didn't understand their mother anymore. She was not the same person they knew and loved when they were younger. It seemed that she picked on them all the time, and that nothing ever pleased her. They felt inadequate and ashamed, because they would do anything to avoid her and stay out of her way. She was too unpredictable for them; she would burst out screaming for almost any incident, and for spilling a glass of milk, one of them might get a severe beating. So they just avoided her.

The ten-year-old felt the brunt of his mother's chronic pain. As the oldest he had more freedom to do something about his situation. After a particularly bad night of pain, Karen started picking on him from the moment he got up until he went to sleep that night. So he ran away. Karen, feeling incapacitated by her pain, just called the police and had him picked up. He was placed in a juvenile facility until Karen came to get him. The ten-year-old ran away several more times—whenever his mother beat him or was especially unpredictable.

Because the father stayed away from home a lot, he was not aware how serious things were for his son. The child spent more time in a state facility than he should have and this had an effect on him. He was unmanageable, unmannerly, and did poorly in school. He said he hated his mother, he did not know why she changed, and he would like to have the old one back; if not, he did not want to live with his parents anymore.

The younger children were also confused and angry. They also didn't like to be near their mother. She had become a malevolent stranger to them, and they preferred to spend time at the homes of their friends. Whenever Karen complained about pain and asked one of them to bring her pills, the youngest would start sucking her thumb and the nine-year-old would hide.

During the therapy session, Karen admitted that she was mortified by her family's behavior and believed that they did not care about her any longer. She had decided that disciplining them was useless, although in the back of her mind, she knew that they needed some firm discipline (dispensed with love).

But she was too fatigued by her pain to discipline, so she yelled and hoped for the best.

Karen's family was falling apart and her pain was responsible.

Her pain made her unpredictable, savagely changing her from a warm (but aggressive) personality into someone who was strange and irritable and highly volatile. She caused her husband to feel angry, guilty and deprived. She confused and overwhelmed her children, and she virtually destroyed herself. Chronic pain was the major cause of the situation in Karen's family.

There is another side to the story of chronic pain and the family. Some families feed on the pain of one of its members. Some families enjoy having someone dependent, someone to cater to, to bring pills to, to feed, to tend to. Such treatment makes the family feel useful and needed. But by doing this the family is keeping the patient in pain by making the pain useful to the patient: his pain becomes a major topic of conversation, a focus of the household duty roster and a way of getting constant attention.

Pain may be useful for the mother who does not want her children to leave the house (and leave her). Pain is useful to the child who does not want to leave the security of his home. Pain can be used to keep a straying husband or a straying wife at home.

Pain can make the whole family sick, which is why pain clinics often recommend that all family members receive treatment. In order to change the patient's attitude toward his pain, the family that contributes to the existence of that attitude also needs treatment. The family attitude must be changed.

# II

## PAIN AND THE PHYSICIAN

*C*hronic pain, you have seen, can work an awful transformation on an ordinarily happy, well-adjusted personality and change it into one that is unrecognizable, unhappy and maybe unlovable. Rarely, however, does the person undergoing this process realize that he is affecting his physician, who has watched him change and has had an almost equal stake in his recovery.

The average physician wants to take care of people and cure them—he's not just a prescription writer, a knee tapper, or someone who refers you to a consultant. He sees himself primarily as a healer, and he is concerned about his patients. Try to imagine, then, what it must be like when a patient who has trusted the doctor with his most prized possession—his health—comes back time after time with the same complaint, still trusting and hoping that the physician can make him better.

When a patient does not respond after repeated attempts by the physician to cure him, the ordinary doctor goes through some changes, too. The physician who is confident about his skills and capabilities, secure in his knowledge that today's medical technology can help or cure almost any ailment, begins to feel inadequate, inept and unskilled when a chronic-pain patient returns again and again, confronting him with his failure. The physician places a lot of the blame for this failure on himself. After all, he put in many years training to be a healer and has been practicing his art for a long time—why can't he help this patient?

Too often, physicians forget that medicine is an art and not yet an exact science. They forget or do not realize that chronic pain is a subjective experience that can't be measured, that can't be forced into quantities or qualities that can be touched, deciphered, rearranged or altered.

Many physicians are unaware of the myriad obscure and hard-to-diagnose diseases that cause chronic pain. So, although the physician wants to help his patient, he is confronted with his own inadequacies and is frustrated in his attempts. This frustration can turn into anxiety for him. After all, he has used all his skills and called upon all the tests known to science (and known to him) to diagnose what seems to be an obvious condition.

After some months the physician eventually asks himself whether the patient's condition could be something that doesn't exist at all. In order to maintain his own confidence and allay his own fears, he comes to the conclusion that the chronic pain is not organic. Since all the tests are negative, since he is unable to relieve it, the chronic pain must be psychosomatic. (Not all physicians come to this conclusion; some stick with the patient for years trying to whip the pain into submission.) In making this diagnosis the physician shifts the responsibility for the patient's condition *from* himself and *onto* the patient. The doctor has decided that if he can't see the pain, if his tests can't measure it, then it simply cannot exist, even if it must be forced out of existence by fiat.

This is not an indictment of those physicians. Most physicians do want to help. What this general conclusion indicates is that chronic pain is a complex, time consuming, elusive disease that can outwit anyone. Chronic pain provokes unpleasant feelings in its victims, and the attending physician eventually becomes a victim too.

The following case focuses on a physician attempting to respond to the problems and crises of a patient afflicted with chronic pain.

> George is a forty-year-old auto mechanic who was injured in a car accident. George did not know that he was injured in any way until two to three days after the accident when he started to feel a sharp pain in the back of his neck that seemed to radiate outward, down his shoulder and right arm.
>
> When the pain started, George went to his family doctor, Morris Smith, whom he had regularly visited for the past twenty years. Morris was a family friend who often went out to dinner with George and his wife on weekends.
>
> Morris was concerned about George and ordered every test he could think of, including an electromyogram, a nerve velocity test, and several other

very sophisticated neurological examinations. All through the testing procedures George tried not to move his arm and shoulder and complained of pain in those areas.

When the test results came back, they were negative. Morris called George back to his office and told him the results. George told him the pain had gotten worse, especially when he tried to use his arm, and that it felt slightly better when he rested his arm on something soft, like a pillow. George confided in Morris that the pain presented something of a problem for him at work because he had to use both hands to be any good at most minor jobs.

Morris talked with George at length and probed for more information. He found out that the damp weather they had the past month also seemed to make George's arm feel worse, but that an application of a heating pad followed by a rubdown (performed by George's wife) made his arm feel a little better.

Morris was worried. George was an old friend who trusted him to seen him through medical problems, and so far he wasn't able to do anything more for George other than tell him to keep on doing the same things that gave him relief. Morris prescribed a painkiller and a sedative and told George to come back to see him in a month if the pain did not get any better.

When George came back the next month, Morris was embarrassed. George complained that the heating pad barely worked anymore and the pain was so incapacitating that he was on the verge of leaving his job.

So Morris recommended that George go to see the best orthopedic surgeon in town. Morris called the surgeon in advance of the appointment to give him George's medical records and he requested that the surgeon please keep him informed as he was very concerned about his patient.

The orthopedic surgeon ran all the tests available and could find nothing out of the ordinary, so he bounced George back to Morris. Morris was getting angry with himself for not being able to help his patient, particularly a patient who was a friend, a friend in pain. Morris thought the pain might even be affecting the friendship.

Morris then suggested that George see a neurosurgeon. George said that he would go if Morris was certain that should be the next step. But he also told Morris that his insurance was running out, he couldn't keep up with the pace at work anymore, and he was going to have to quit. He was thinking of applying for Social Security disability payments, but his wife was reluctant. She couldn't face her friends if she felt that they knew she and her husband were on "welfare." Morris was upset when he heard that. He was also feeling helpless because all he could do was to recommend this second consultation—it resulted in the neurosurgeon sending George on to a neurologist who also found nothing.

Meanwhile, the Social Security board, in reviewing George's application, sent George back to three more doctors: an orthopedic surgeon, a neurologist and a neurosurgeon. Though they were different people from the first three specialists he had consulted, they all told him the same thing.

During all his visits to physicians, George from time to time called Morris to tell him about the latest reviews his pain received. Morris was already aware of all the consultation results, as the physicians had all called him to obtain George's medical records.

By now Morris was beginning to feel suspicious. He began to think that if seven physicians could find nothing wrong with George, perhaps, in fact, nothing was wrong.

Morris decided that George probably was faking the pain in order to get the disability payments and therefore have an excuse to retire. He just could no longer believe that something was wrong. He had done his best, and now he felt that George, perhaps, was using him, or that possibly the pain was all in George's head. He preferred to think that rather than to think that his friend was using him.

Finally, Morris referred George to an anesthesiologist who specialized in nerve blocks. After performing several tests, the anesthesiologist told him that he was not a suitable candidate for a nerve block.

George ended his odyssey in Morris's office. But Morris was no longer prepared to deal with his pain. George represented a mystery to him, as well as a failure. Since he could not cure him, perhaps, he thought, a psychiatrist could; and that is what he told George, though not exactly in those words. George was angry and left Morris's office feeling resentful, but he went to see the psychiatrist.

After evaluating George's psychological history, the psychiatrist decided that he was not a malingerer. He ordered a thermography test and found that there was an area of pain in his shoulders. He decided to test George for myofascial syndrome by pressing on two trigger points in the area that he complained about. George yelped in pain. The psychiatrist explained that feeling the pain at the trigger points indicated that he was probably a victim of primary myofascial syndrome. George was relieved to know that his pain was "real" after all, even though so many doctors had implied that the pain did not really exist.

What about Morris; how did he feel? By the time Morris sent George to the psychiatrist, he was feeling inept, inadequate, embarrassed and confused. If George ever returned to his office, Morris knew their relationship could never be the same. George represented failure to him. George probably knew how desperately Morris wanted to cure him and probably will not return to Morris, who, it seems, loses on all counts.

Most physicians are similar to Morris in that they try their best to heal or cure their patients and see failure to heal or cure as a personal and professional disaster. (There is, however, one kind of chronic-pain patient who is offensive to the physician. This is the malingerer, as described in Chapter 5. The malingerer, who consciously tries to deceive the doctor for his own personal gain, can make the most patient physician lost control and objectivity.) Chronic-pain patients always present a challenge, but they also are symbols of potential failure and for this reason may frighten some physicians.

# 12

## WHAT PRICE RELIEF?

*I*t is not at all unusual for a victim of chronic pain to spend $50,000 or more seeking relief from his affliction.

This dollar figure accounts for doctors' fees, drugs, surgery and hospital bed space, psychiatric bills, travel and so on, but it does not measure how much is spent in time and personal energy, nor does it consider the cost borne by the patient's family.

How much you will spend in a pain clinic is impossible to estimate with any accuracy, and it would be irresponsible of me or anyone else unfamiliar with the particulars of an individual's situation to try. The costs vary widely from city to city and coast to coast and are subject to change at any time.

Another factor that will influence greatly the total cost you'll incur at a pain clinic is the amount your insurance company will pick up.

Your insurance plan might pay for most of a pain

clinic stay, depending on the type of services you receive. You have to examine your insurance policy to determine whether or not you can be reimbursed for services and physicians' fees. It's important to remember that while recommended prescription items may not be paid for, your prescription bill is likely to be reduced rather than increased when you are finished with your treatment at the pain clinic. Talk to the insurance company to find out what they will pay for; it never hurts to ask, and you may be surprised at how much is covered. Also, it may be useful to discuss financial arrangements with the pain clinic staff. These people often have experience with the many different insurance carriers, and they may be able to help you decipher exactly what benefits are due to you.

If you are eligible, Medicaid and Medicare will pick up some of the costs of a pain-treatment center. Medicare will pay for some clinical services and some of the electrical stimulator devices. Medicaid payment varies, according to what each state's plan picks up as optional services. Again, inquire from the local board before checking into the clinic.

Regardless of the cost of the chronic-pain-treatment center, we can only offer the following advice. Seek out chronic-pain-treatment facilities with academic affiliations. Also, find a center that uses a multi-disciplinary approach to the diagnosis and treatment of chronic pain, and be wary of any pain clinic that makes exaggerated claims for success. Avoid any clinic that uses a single modality of treatment for all types of pain or that fails to provide any diagnostic evaluation prior to beginning treatment. Check the credentials of the physicians who are associated with the chronic-pain-treatment center—this may be done through the *Marquis Compendium of Medical Specialists*. If a physician is listed in this reference text, this means he has been certified by the medical board in his specialty and has exhibited a degree of competence within a given field. This does not imply that physicians who are not board certified are not qualified, or that those who are certified are qualified, but it certainly does provide some guideline when seeking medical attention. Avoid any chronic-pain-treatment center that advocates the use of narcotics, analgesics, hypnotics or sedative drugs. There is no pharmacological rationale for the use of these drugs in the treatment of chronic pain, unless it is intractable cancer pain. The physician who subscribes to this therapy is not as well-informed as he should be about the treatment of chronic pain.

# A List of Pain Clinics

The following is a partial list of pain clinics in the United States. These are by no means all the clinics, but the list does represent most of the best multi-disciplinary pain-treatment centers. For more information, and to locate the clinic nearest you, contact your local medical society or the Committee on Accreditation of Rehabilitation Facilities (CARF).

Boston Pain Unit
Massachusetts General Hospital
Boston, MA 02114

Cleveland Clinic
9500 Euclid Avenue
Cleveland, OH 44195

Cox Pain Center
San Luis Obispo, CA 93401

Emory Clinic Pain Control Center
Emory University
Atlanta, GA 30333

Johns Hopkins University School of Medicine
Pain Treatment Center
Baltimore, MD 21205

Mayo Clinic
200 SW First Street
Rochester, MN 55905

Medical Center
Del Oro Hospital
Houston, TX 77002

Mensana Clinic
1718 Greenspring Valley Road
Stevenson, MD 21153

Mount Sinai Hospital
Pain Consultation Center
Miami, FL 33101

New York Pain Treatment Program
Lenox Hill Hospital
New York, NY

New York University Medical Center School of Medicine
New York, NY 10016

Pain Control and Rehabilitation Institute of Georgia
3375 Holcomb Bridge Road
Norcross, GA 30092

Rush Presbyterian-St. Luke's Medical Center Pain Clinic
Chicago, IL 60607

Scripps Clinic
Pain Treatment Center
Claremont, CA 91711

University of California-Los Angeles
Pain Control Unit
Los Angeles, CA 90024

University of Illinois School of Medicine
Pain Clinic
Chicago, IL 60612

University of Miami School of Medicine
Pain Evaluation Team
Miami, FL 33101

University of Pittsburgh Pain Control Center
Pittsburgh, PA 15261

University of Washington School of Medicine
Pain Clinic
Seattle, WA 98195

# GLOSSARY

**acetaminophen (Tylenol):** a chemical that can reduce pain and fever, but does not have the anti-inflammatory properties of aspirin.

**acetylcholine:** one of the neurosynaptic transmitters. This chemical is located in the brain and the parasympathetic system. Like norepinephrine (see below) it has specific receptors in blood vessels, nerves and muscles. The action of acetylcholine usually is antagonistic to the action of norepinephrine.

**acupuncture:** the insertion of needles in and around the nerve, producing numbness in the surrounding area. The **analgesia:** a loss of the sensation of pain.

**addiction:** a physiological state in which a person develops a tolerance to a particular drug and needs ever-increasing dosages of the drug to obtain the same effect. Also, when the drug is no longer taken, the person experiences "withdrawal" symptoms, which indicate the existence of a physical dependence on this chemical. This reaction is found with opiates, barbiturates and benzodiazepines.

**adhesion:** a band of fiber-like material on the surface of a membrane that connects to the surface of another membrane, as an adhesion between one side of a wound and another.

**analgesia:** a loss of the sensation of pain.

**analgesic:** any compound that relieves pain without producing anesthesia or loss of consciousness.

**anesthesia:** generally a state characterized by a loss of any sensation caused by the depression of nerve function either with drugs or by disease.

**anesthesiologist:** a physician who specializes in the administration of chemicals that produce a sleep-like state with some reduction of pain sensation for patients prior to operations. Also, these physicians are skilled and trained in injecting various areas of the body to produce pain relief.

**antidepressant:** any chemical that relieves the feeling of depression.

**antihistamine:** the body contains histamine, which causes a variety of symptoms, such as runny nose, red eyes and excessive mucous formation. Any medication that blocks the action of histamine is called an antihistamine.

**anxiety:** a dread or fear of danger that can be accompanied by tension, restlessness or palpitations; usually there is no clearly identifiable reason for these feelings of apprehension.

**arthritis:** a medical disease that may be caused by a local inflammation in a joint, damage to the joint itself, or infection. There are a number of different forms of this disease, variously called rheumatoid, osteo and gonorrheal arthritis. Any inflammation of a joint is an arthritis.

**atrophy:** a reduction in size of a muscle group due to lack of use, which may occur either on a voluntary or involuntary basis (see paralysis).

**axon:** the part of the cell that conducts nervous impulses to dendrites away from the body cell. The axon looks somewhat like a filament and varies in thickness and length, up to fifty centimeters long.

**axonal:** pertaining to a nerve axon. A nerve axon is the long, pipe-like tube that connects the cell body at one end to the terminal ending that contains neurosynaptic transmitters.

**barbiturate:** a drug that is a central nervous system depressant; it slows down the activities of the central nervous system.

**behavior modification:** a psychological technique by which a form of behavior is altered, without regard to the motivation that has produced it. In this technique, analogous to training a dog or a cat, a series of psychological maneuvers, such as the dispensing of rewards and punishment and the shaping of behavior, are used.

**benzodiazepines:** a group of chemicals that are the "minor tranquilizers" and are the most prescribed drugs in the United States today. These produce anxiety reduction, but may create addiction, dependence and a variety of other undesirable side effects, including depression.

**biofeedback:** a technique by which certain body functions, such as temperature and muscle tension, which a person cannot measure by himself, are measured for him by an instrument and "fed back" to him. By virtue of this ability to visualize bodily functions, a person can then gain control over functions that he previously could not control.

**block:** arresting the passage of a nervous impulse usually by injecting a chemical, either alcohol or a local anesthetic solution, directly into the nerve.

**Briquet's syndrome:** people with Briquet's syndrome usually have a variety of minor physical complaints, but because they generally have had moderate to severe psychiatric difficulties beforehand, they are overwhelmed by these difficulties and dwell on them.

**bursitis:** an inflammation of the sac covering a joint (the sac contains a fluid that lubricates the joint). When this covering is inflamed, it produces a syndrome that may be mistaken for arthritis, but is in actuality bursitis. It is usually accompanied by swelling and increased fluid in the area around the joint.

**CAT or tomographic scan:** a test that takes a multiple group of X-rays from a variety of angles, and provides a three-dimensional view of certain areas under investigation. This has replaced several painful and sometimes dangerous tests.

**causalgia:** a severe persistent burning sensation in the skin normally following an injury, either direct or indirect, to the sensory fibers of a peripheral nerve.

**classical conditioning:** in this technique, described by Pavlov, an animal or human is trained to respond to a stimulus to which he normally would not react. He eventually begins to respond to what previously had been a neutral stimulus with almost the same degree of intensity as he responds to a natural stimulus. The standard example of this process was Pavlov's pairing of the sound of a bell with the presentation of food in order to get a dog to salivate. In time, the sound of the bell alone was enough to induce salivation.

**dementia:** a loss of memory and the ability to reason which may be caused by a variety of problems, such as old age, with concomitant blockage of blood vessels to the brain. In this case, it is called senile dementia. Alcohol, other chemical substances, vitamin deficiencies and some neurological diseases may cause other types of dementia.

**dendrite:** a branch of a nerve cell that receives nerve impulses from the axon of a neighboring nerve.

**denervation:** an operation that cuts off the nerve supply to a particular part of the body by incision, excision, blocking or burning the nerve.

**depression:** a dejected feeling where the person feels so bad or low that it is readily discernible to others. Depressions are either reactive (in response to a situation such as the lost of a loved one) or endogenous (coming from within and having no discernible external cause such as the loss mentioned above).

**dopamine:** a neurosynaptic transmitter usually found in the brain that is specifically associated with some forms of psychosis and abnormal movement disorders. This chemical also causes vessels to constrict.

**dystrophy:** literally means defective nutrition. Sympathetic reflex dystrophy refers to a painful illness that has a spreading or burning sensation, usually occurs in a limb, and leads to a restriction in motion in the affected limb. Trauma is a major cause of sympathetic reflex dystrophy.

**electrical stimulators:** see transcutaneous stimulators.

**electromyographic:** refers to the measurement of the electrical component of muscle action. Every time a nerve sends information to the muscle to make it move, an electrical impulse travels down the nerve, causing the release of a chemical. The electrical impulse can be measured by a variety of instruments such as biofeedback instruments and machines.

**endorphin:** a naturally produced chemical that has a morphine-like action and is usually found in the brain. High concentrations of endorphin are believed to cause the relief of pain and may be the body's own protection against pain.

**enkephalin:** like endorphin, a naturally produced chemical that has a morphine-like action. Enkephalin is usually found in the brain and the spinal cord, and its action is analogous to endorphin's action.

**etiology:** the cause of a disease.

**euphoria:** a feeling or sensation of well-being, Sometimes an exaggerated feeling of being on top of the world physically as well as emotionally.

**facet:** a small smooth area on a bone, or a place that has been worn away on a smooth, firm structure.

**facet blocks:** a test done either by an anesthesiologist or a neurosurgeon, in which a numbing substance (local anesthetic) is injected in and around a nerve found on the bony surface of the vertebrae in the back. In some instances this injection can reduce or eliminate some painful syndromes of the back.

**fascia:** covering over the muscle that allows it to glide over adjacent muscle.

**gate theory:** an attempt to explain the mechanism by which the sensation of pain is reduced through the intentional irritation of areas in the same nerve distribution as the sensation. Basically, it says that if you overload a pathway, it will not be able to transmit all the messages it receives and will selectively decide to eliminate the painful transmission.

**generic:** the non-trademark name for a drug; its class.

**housemaid's knee:** a form of bursitis (see above) that is caused by repeated injury (such as constant kneeling) to the covering of the knee joint.

**hypnosis:** a repetitive series of statements that alters the attention of its subject and makes him extremely receptive to suggestions.

**hypnotic:** any chemical that, after administration, allows the person to sleep.

**hysterical conversion:** an unconscious defense against a horrible psychological trauma. In most cases the patient is overwhelmed or overcome by something they have thought, seen or experienced. In order to cope with this trauma, the patient develops a symptom, such as blindness, paralysis or spasm, which then can account for the severity of his reaction.

**iatrogenic:** resulting from the administrations or activities of a physician or surgeon.

**innervation:** the actual supply of nerve fibers to a particular part of the body.

**ischemia:** a reduced blood flow to part of the body.

**keloid:** an overgrowth of scar tissue that far exceeds the normal growth of scar tissue for a given injury.

**Lamaze method:** a technique for assisting childbirth that consists of informing the mother of the various stages of delivery prior to the onset of labor and instructing both parents in a routine that has hypnotic-like qualities. The result is the reduction of the anxiety and pain associated with childbirth.

**lesion:** a wound or injury, or any change in tissue.

**limbic system:** an area in the brain associated with the control of emotion, eating, drinking and sexual activity.

**MMPI (Minnesota Multiphasic Personality Inventory):** a 566-question test that asks true-false questions. The patient takes this test himself, and then a psychologist scores it and interprets personality characteristics.

**monoamine oxidase:** an enzyme found in the nerve endings that breaks down certain neurosynaptic transmitters, such as serotonin, norepinephrine and dopamine. By blocking this chemical with the use of monoamine oxidase inhibitors, an accumulation of these neurosynaptic transmitters can occur.

**monoamine oxidase inhibitors:** a group of chemicals used to treat depression, in some instances phobic anxiety, and may have some limited application in the treatment of pain. (See above.)

**multi-disciplinary pain-treatment center:** a pain-treatment center where the emphasis is placed on diagnosis of the origin of the painful syndrome. This involves the input of a variety of physicians, including neurosurgeon, neurologists, orthopedic surgeons, anesthesiologists, psychiatrists, psychologists, and, on occasion, rheumatoidologists, internists, and endocrinologists. After the diagnosis has been established, treatment is begun in a two-prong fashion—treatment of the physical causes and effects of pain and an effort to help the person deal with the psychological problems caused by the pain.

**muscle guarding:** when an area of the body is damaged, there is an involuntary response called muscle guarding that manifests itself as increased muscle tension over the injured area.

**myelin:** a protein-like material that envelops the axons of nerve fibers. It is composed of alternating layers of fats (lipid) and proteins. Myelin is analogous to the insulation on an electrical wire, allowing electrical impulses to remain within the nerve bundle without spreading to adjacent nerves.

**myofascial syndrome:** *myo* means muscle and *fascial* means the covering over the muscle that is very smooth and allows one muscle group to glide freely across another muscle group. When the muscle is damaged by an injury to the body, blood and other substances get into the space between muscles that is separated by the fascial covering. A scar, or an adhesion, is then formed in this area and the muscles are prevented from gliding smoothly over one another. The result is muscle spasm, and later, pain.

**narcotic:** any substance producing a stupor-like state while it kills pain; more specifically, a drug derived from opium or opium-like compounds that can affect mood and behavior and has a potential for dependence and tolerance.

**nerve:** a whitish cord made up of fibers arranged in bundles and held together with connective tissue (myelin).

**neuralgia:** nerve pain that feels like severe throbbing or stabbing along the nerve pathway.

**neuritis:** an inflammation of a nerve that may be caused by a viral infection, mechanical irritation or reduced blood flow. This may manifest as a burning sensation, exquisite increase in sensitivity, paralysis, numbness or muscular atrophy in areas of the body (skin and muscle) supplied by the nerve.

**neuroleptic:** any chemical that can serve as a tranquilizer with specific antipsychotic actions is called a neuroleptic. This is a category of drugs, rather than one specific drug.

**neuroma:** when a nerve is crushed as the result of an injury, a number of chemicals are released that help it to regenerate and restore its function. However, the injury usually destroys the channels through which the nerve should grow, so that sensory nerves, especially pain nerves, develop into a tangled, bird's nest pattern. This mass of tangle of free nerve endings is called a neuroma, and is exquisitely painful to the touch.

**neuron:** the nerve cell.

**neurosis:** a psychological or behavior disorder in which anxiety plays a prime part. People with neuroses do not necessarily exhibit a gross distortion of reality; more often they have phobias or are unable to cope with stress situations.

**neurosynaptic transmitter:** same as a neurotransmitter.

**neurotransmitter:** a chemical released by the pre-synaptic cell that crosses the synapse to inhibit or excite the post-synaptic cell.

**norepinephrine:** one of the neurosynaptic transmitters, this chemical is found in the brain and in the endings of some sympathetic nerves. There are specific receptors for norepinephrine located in a variety of tissue such as the blood vessels, nerves and specialized muscles like the heart. Sometimes the blocking of this chemical can reduce pain sensations.

**normal:** healthy according to a standard.

**operant conditioning:** this is a technique developed by Thorndike, and expanded by Skinner, by which animals and humans (see behavior modification above) can be trained to do certain tasks by using a system based on the meting out of rewards and punishment and the shaping of behavior. The important factor here is the use of a reward when a desired behavior is achieved.

**organic:** related to the body (as opposed to the mind), such as a disease that is organic in origin; that is, starting in or caused by some organ (any part of the body that has a specific function).

**opiate:** any chemical derived from opium that produces pain relief and a state of well-being.

**palatal myoclonus:** this very rare syndrome is caused by damage to specific motor centers in the brain stem (the lower portion of the brain). It is manifested as a spasmodic contraction in the soft palate, located at the upper-rear portion of the mouth.

**paleospinothalamic tract:** an area in the spinal cord that runs alongside the neospinothalamic tract and becomes active when painful stimulation is constant and chronic (lasting longer than six months). This tract reaches areas in the brain in addition to the thalamus, eventually involving areas of the hypothalamus and limbic system, thereby creating the emotional components associated with chronic pain.

**paralysis:** the loss of power or voluntary control over the use of a muscle due to injury or disease of its nerve supply. The damage may occur anywhere along the pathway from the brain, spinal cord, specific nerve, or the junction between the nerve and muscle. This may result in atrophy of the muscle due to disuse.

**paranoia:** a mental disorder marked by delusions that the person is being persecuted and that he is special. Often a paranoid personality has an otherwise normal grasp of reality.

**percutaneous rhizotomy:** the permanent destruction of a nerve coming from the spinal cord that carries the sensory fibers from a particular area of skin and muscle. The procedure involves the insertion of a needle through the skin and muscle to the nerve to be destroyed, using an X-ray-like device (fluoroscope) for direct visualization and the application of electrical current to burn away the sensory component of the nerve.

**phantom limb pain:** when an appendage, such as an arm or leg, has been traumatically amputated, very often the person will continue to report a sensation of pain, itching or burning in the missing limb. This indicates that the brain is still receiving messages from the severed nerve fibers and is interpreting them as if the limb were still present.

**phenothiazines:** a group of tranquilizers, or neuroeleptics, that are specifically used for the treatment of psychoses. At lower dosages they can be useful for the treatment of anxiety and, in some instances, for the treatment of pain states, since they interfere with the chemicals that transmit painful messages.

**phlebogram:** a test in which dye is injected into the venous system, and photographs (a series of X-rays) are taken in order to ascertain whether there is any obstruction in the veins.

**placebo effect:** anytime a substance or activity can produce a desired result without the use of what is considered an active agent, this is termed a placebo effect. This phenomenon is poorly understood, but basically indicates that a patient who receives attention, regardless of the type of medication or manipulation administered, will derive benefit from the personal contact.

**pleurisy:** just as the muscles have a covering called the fascia, the lungs have a covering known as the pleura. When this covering is inflamed, breathing becomes painful. Any inflammation of the pleura is called pleurisy.

**post-herpetic neuralgia:** any irritation or inflammation of a nerve that is the result of an infection that is caused by the herpes virus. The most common post-herpetic neuralgia is herpes zoster (shingles) and trigeminal neuralgia.

**psychoanalysis:** a method of psychotherapy originated by Sigmund Freud in the nineteenth century that attempts to bring unconscious or subconscious material to the patient's conscious, then analyze it for therapeutic benefit.

**psychogenic:** of mental origin; related to psychic processes of behavior, personality and other psychological processes.

**psychosis:** a mental disorder affecting a person's organization of thoughts, perception of reality, ability to communicate with other people, and capacity to cope with daily stresses and demands. Psychoses may be caused by severe emotional stress, biochemical abnormalities in the brain, or the natural aging process, resulting in organic brain syndromes. Certain drugs also may induce psychoses.

**psychostimulants:** a group of chemicals that excite the entire brain. Caffeine and amphetamine-like substances may be included in this group.

**receptor:** a specialized area on a nerve membrane, a blood vessel or a muscle, which receives the chemical stimulation that activates or inhibits the nerve, blood vessel or muscle.

**reflex sympathetic dystrophy:** a disorder of the sympathetic nervous system, due to either entrapment or damage. The critical manifestations are tingling, pins and needles sensations, and coldness in the affected limb. In extreme forms, hair loss and loss of bone from the fingertips or toetips is visible on X-rays. This disorder can easily be detected with the use of thermography.

**schizophrenia:** the most common type of psychosis, characterized by delusions, hallucinations, and a withdrawal from relationships with other people into a world of one's own. Schizophrenia is thought to be a group of disorders rather than a single illness.

**SCL 90-R:** this is a test very similar to the MMPI (see MMPI above), but it contains only 90 questions compared to the MMPI's 566. This test also has the capacity to measure changes in the person's response over time, which the MMPI does not.

**sedative:** any chemical that calms a person down: it also produces drowsiness.

**sensation:** the translation of a stimulus into a consciousness of the effects of the stimulus; a feeling.

**serotonin:** a chemical found in the brain and in some areas of the intestine, as well as in circulating blood. There are receptors for this chemical in the brain associated with the relief of depression, in the vessel walls associated with an intense constriction of the vessel, and in the intestines associated with increased bowel motility.

**somatogenic:** a disorder or disease with clear-cut physical origins. *Soma* means body and *genic* is a term for arising from.

**spinothalamic tract:** an area in the spinal cord that transmits pain messages from the skin and muscles to the area of the brain that receives painful inputs.

**steroid:** a class of chemicals sharing a common structure that almost always function as hormones. These hormones are produced by the glands, including the ovaries or testicles and the adrenal gland.

**sympathetic nerve blocks:** in several painful syndromes (reflect sympathetic dystrophy), a numbing injection in the area of the sympathetic nerves may produce relief. If this is done repeatedly permanent relief may sometimes be obtained from a variety of the painful syndromes.

**synapse:** the gap between the membrane of one nerve cell and the membrane of another. The synapse is the point at which the transmission of nerve impulses occurs.

**syndrome:** the combination of signs and symptoms of a morbid process that constitutes a disease.

**temporomandibular joint:** a joint located between the bones of the skull and the lower jaw. This is the most unusual joint in the human body—the only one that can move in three directions: side to side; forward and back in a gliding fashion; in a hinge-like opening motion. Damage to this joint, either by excessive grinding of the teeth (bruxism), or by injury to the muscle attaching the jaw to the skull (myofascial syndrome) can create a painful syndrome called temporomandibular joint syndrome.

**tennis elbow:** the result of repeated injury to the ligaments and tendons that hold the elbow joints together. This may be tendinitis, or, in some cases, an arthritis. This is due to repeated injury to a joint by excessive use.

**thalamus:** an area in the brain that receives pain messages from the spinothalamic tract and sends these messages to the cortex, which allows the perception and realization of pain.

**thermocoagulation:** the technique employed for performing a percutaneous rhizotomy. This means the application of a high temperature probe, usually produced by the passage of electrical current, which selectively burns away the smaller sensory or pain carrying nerves, leaving the larger, motor nerves intact.

**thermography:** a specialized test to detect temperature differences caused by cancer growth or by injuries to the nervous system or blood vessels. Using heat-sensitive detection devices, a photograph may be taken in which the damaged area shows up as either warmer (in the case of cancer) or colder (in the case of pain that is caused by damaged vessels) than the rest of the body.

**tic douloureux:** a painful and sometimes disabling syndrome accompanied by horribly sharp shooting pains in the face. This is a synonym for trigeminal neuralgia.

**transcutaneous stimulators:** devices that emit an electrical current, which takes away certain types of pain. They are small devices that can be worn continuously and are available from a variety of sources.

**trauma:** an injury caused by rough contact with a physical object; an accidental or inflicted wound.

**tricyclic antidepressants:** a group of chemicals that are used to treat depression and, in some instances, to treat chronic pain.

**trigeminal neuralgia:** an irritation of the fifth cranial nerve, one of the nerves in the face. This irritation is usually caused by either a mechanical abrasion of the nerve or by a viral infection. This is also called tic douloureux.

# BIBLIOGRAPHY

Adolphe, Allen B., Ph.D.; Dorsey, Richard E., M.D.; Napoliello, Michael J., M.D. "Neuropharmacology of Depression." *Diseases of the Nervous System.* 38(1977):841–46.

Axelrod, Julius. "Neurotransmitters." *Scientific American.* 230(1974):58–71.

Beecher, H.K. "Relationship of Significant Wounds to Pain." *Journal of the American Medical Association.* 161(1956):1607–13.

Breuer, Josef, and Freud, Sigmund. "On the Psychical Mechanisms of Hysterical Phenomena." *Preliminary Communication (1893) in Studies on Hysteria.* New York: Avon Books, 1966, pp. 37–52.

Brown, Burnell, Jr., M.D., Ph.D. "Diagnosis and Therapy of Common Myofascial Syndromes." *Journal of the American Medical Association.* 239(1978):2386–89.

*Drugs of Abuse*, 4th ed. Washington, D.C. U.S. Dept. of Justice, Drug Enforcement Administration, 1977. Produced by the Office of Public Affairs in Cooperation with the Office of Science and Technology.

Eccles, Sir John. "The Synapse." *Scientific American.* 212(1965): 52–66.

Freud, Sigmund. "Fixation upon Trauma: The Unconscious." *A General Introduction to Psychoanalysis*. New York: Washington Square Press, 1963, pp. 284–96.

Funt, Lawrence, D.D.S., M.S., and Stack, Brendon, D.D.S., M.S. "The Evolution of the Craniomandibular Pain Syndrome, F.S. Index." *Clinical Management of Head, Neck and T.M.J. Pain and Dysfunction*. Edited by Harold Gelb. Philadelphia: W. B. Saunders Company, 1978.

Gehris, C. W., Jr., M.D.; Hendler, Nelson, M.D. "Myoclonus Presenting as a Pulsatile Neck Mass." A paper presented at the eighty-first annual meeting of the American Academy of Ophthalmology and Otolaryngology, 6–10 October 1976, at Las Vegas.

"The Great Imposter: Diseases of the Temporomandibular Joint." *Journal of the American Medical Association*. Commentary. 235(1976): 2395.

Hancock, Elise. "To Sleep: Perchance to Dream." *Johns Hopkins Magazine*. 84(1977): 29–35.

Hendler, Nelson H., M.D. "Group Therapy with Pain Patients." Chapter 15 in *Diagnosis and Non-Surgical Management of Chronic Pain*. New York: Raven Press, 1979.

—. "Psychiatric Considerations of Pain." Chapter 104 in *Textbook of Neurosurgery*. Edited by J. Youmans, M.D., Ph.D. Philadelphia: W. B. Saunders Company, 1979.

—. "Psychopharmacology of Chronic Pain." Chapter 14 in *Diagnosis and Non-Surgical Management of Chronic Pain*. New York: Raven Press, 1979.

—. "Psychiatric Considerations of Pain." Chapter 116 in *Neurological Surgery*, edited by Julian Youmans, M.D., Ph.D., W. B. Saunders Co., Philadelphia, 1982, pp. 3480–3522.

—. "Drug Therapy in Chronic Pain.", Chapter 316, in *Neurosurgery*, edited by Robert Wilkins, M.D. and Setti Rengachary, M.D., McGraw-Hill, New York, 1985, pp. 2374–2381.

—. "Psychotherapy." Chapter 34, in *Principles and Practice of Pain Management*, edited by Carol Warfield, M.D., McGraw-Hill, New York, 1993, pp 455–466.

Hendler, Nelson, M.D.; Derogatis, Leonard, Ph.D.; Avella, Jane, B.S.; Long, Donlin, M.D., Ph.D. "EMG Biofeedback in Patients with Chronic Pain." *Diseases of the Nervous System*. 39(1977):505–9.

Hendler, Nelson, M.D.; Long, Donlin, M.D., Ph.D.; Black, Richard, M.D.; and Vernstein, Mary, Ph.D. "Diagnostic Screening Test for Chronic Pain Patients: A Selection Process for Surgery and Other Treatment Procedures." A paper presented at the second International Congress on Pain, August 1978, at Montreal.

Hendler, Nelson, M.D.; Wise, Tom, M.D.; and Lucas, Jane, R.N. "Expanded Role of the Psychiatric Nurse." A paper presented at the annual American Psychiatric Association meeting, May 1977, at Toronto. (Accepted for publication in *Psychiatric Quarterly*.)

Hendler, Nelson, M.D., and Talo, Seija, Ph.L.: *Role of The Pain Clinic, in Current Therapy of Pain*, edited by Kathy Foley, M.D., and Richard Payne, M.D., B.C. Decker, Toronto, 1989, pp 23–32.

Keiser, Lester, M.D. *The Traumatic Neuroses*. Philadelphia: J. B. Lippincott Company, 1968, chap. 13.

Kubler-Ross, Elisabeth, M.D. *On Death and Dying*. New York: Macmillan, Inc., 1969.

Melzak, P., and Chapman, C. R. "Psychological Aspects of Pain." *Postgraduate Medicine*. 53(1973): 69–75.

Synder, Solomon H., M.D. "Opiate Receptors and Internal Opiates." *Scientific American*. 236(1977):44–56.

Sternbach, Richard. *Pain Patients' Traits and Treatments*. New York: Academic Press, 1974.

Uematsu, Sumio, M.D.; Long, Donlin, M.D., Ph.D. "Thermography in Chronic Pain." *Medical Thermography, Theory and Clinical Applications*. Edited by Sumio Uematsu, M.D. Los Angeles: Brentwood Publishing Corp., 1976, pp. 52–67.

Whistler, W. D., and Hill, B.J. "A Simplified Technique for Inspection of the Gasserian Ganglion." *Treatment of Pain*. Edited by Harold Voris, M.D., Ph.D., and Walter Whistler, M.D., Ph.D. Springfield, Illinois: Charles C. Thomas Publisher, 1975, pp. 61–74.

# INDEX